Sorgitzak: Old Forest Craft

Sorgitzak: Old Forest Craft

by

Veronica Cummer

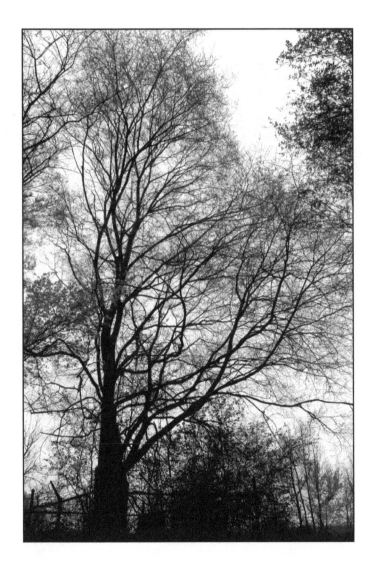

PENDRAIG PUBLISHING, LOS ANGELES

Pendraig Publishing, Sunland, CA 91040
© Veronica Cummer 2008. All rights reserved.
Published 2008.
Printed in the United States of America

ISBN 978-0-9796168-6-0

Contents

Dedication

Many thanks to those who once walked and who still walk this Path with me. To those who came and showed us what once was and what could be, be they spirit, God, or Witch. This book is dedicated to you.

It is dedicated to those who never lost faith, and to those who did. To those who chose to follow the light and those who chose to fall into darkness. In the completion of the circle may the two worlds meet once more in the fullness of time.

To Giahna, who opened the door and to Ardwena who first walked in. *Gobah*. To the gracious Muse, whose beauty and strength always inspires and without whom these words would be sadly lacking, if even here at all. Blessings and praise to you, Ariadne.

This work is also dedicated to those who were comforting and to those who were strict, each when it was most needed. To those who spoke in riddles or in plain unvarnished truth, though it was sometimes painful to hear. To those who came and laughed with us and cried with us, and showed us the two weren't all that dissimilar. To those who came before and to those who shall come after. Blessings be upon all of you.

Nothing is ever truly lost, so long as we remember.

PREFACE

One candle is lit, two, a third, and then a fourth. We make our world. We make our worlds. A blade is raised, two, a third, and then many. We call the powers to our circle, four powers, eight, sixteen, each one a world.

How many times have we walked this way? How many times more? To wake the powers, to raise the circle, to send out a light into the greater darkness...

We step through the door and it changes us. We walk in the outer darkness, each bringing the light. Together, we make a court upon the hill, a circle of candles. Together, we make a starry crown.

What will we leave behind, for those who come after, if not a touch of the light?

This book is a work of many years. It has its source and its beginning in revealed knowledge. Through contact with and channeled messages from many of the Gods and Goddesses of the *Sorgitza*, through those who have come to be called the Fey, as well as other spirits and entities, much has been remembered and much has been recovered. There yet remains a great deal to be explored and reclaimed, as is ever befitting of Mystery. In many cases, it is not the right answers that we must first seek out, but the right questions.

The Gods and Goddesses of this pantheon have graced many Priests and Priestesses with Their presence, as well as with Their love and guidance, over the past dozen or more years and we have learned from each and every experience. Through Their words and by what They have taught us, the experiences They have shared with us, we have glimpsed the world of Witches long past and have begun the task of understanding once again—what was lost, what might be found, and what never truly left us.

This book is but a step along the way and one freely encouraged by the Gods and Goddesses found herein. They wish to be known again as of old, to be remembered, and to be with those of us who are called to Them, to Their service and to Their love. All religion begins in this way—through direct and intimate contact with the Divine.

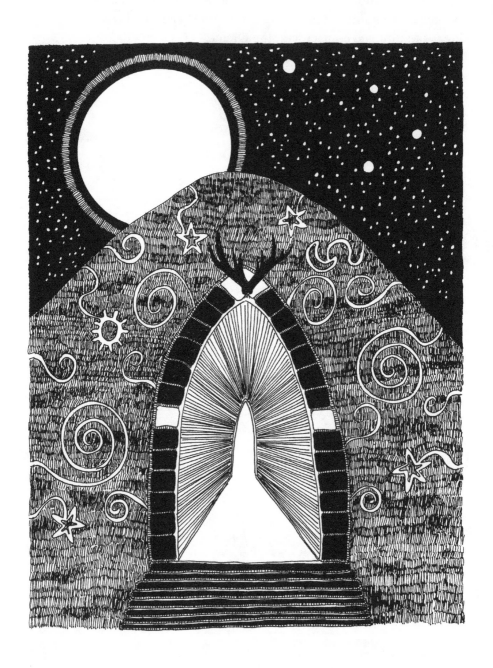

Introduction
To Not Forget

*Ancient of days, the ways of the Sorgitza came to be. Descended of the stars
and bound to the earth, for the love of the earth they stayed and walked among the
ancestors and descendants of man.*

*Sorgitza are those who know they are yet spirit. That they are of the starry heavens
and that the fire of those stars, the fire of heaven, burns yet in their bones and in their
blood. Sorgitza are those who remember the dance, and in the dance, they remember.*

A Legend from the Fey

Orahno ze zomah
Orahno ze arhanahk
Arhanahk itzah
Arhanahk ahzarah

This is a book of the Old Religion. This is a book of the Old Ways.

Here within you will find the Gods of the Old Ones, Witches of the Blood,
the *Sorgitza* who once lived in the Old Forest, the great haunted woodlands
which used to cover most of Europe and of which a few small lingering
pockets yet remain. The *Sorgitza* existed in secret places in what is now
France, Spain, Germany, Switzerland, all the way to Romania, Poland, and
Hungary. Though, of course, these lands were not known by those names
in years long past.

A few of these Witch Gods have been asleep for countless generations,
some since before the rise of the Roman Empire. Others of them have
been awake, but almost forgotten, their altars and faith left untended and

all but unknown. Some of their beliefs have been lost within the mists of an age so long ago that only a few remnants have come to be passed down to us today, much of which is confusing or misleading to say the least.

These Gods are part of an old European Witch pantheon, one based upon the elements and the directions of the circle. North, South, East, West, the center, and the rim, and so much more between. It is now, at the dawning of the Age of the Water-Bearer, the Age of Aquarius, that the Old Gods have returned and are speaking to us, teaching us of what has been lost, we who are the children and the children's children of those once known and beloved of Them. The Wheel has turned and so They have returned to us as we have returned to Them.

Sadly, though, much has been lost of the culture of the Old Ones, the ancient Witches, in part due to the long passage of years, but also due to the efforts of conquering peoples and religions. If a lot has simply been forgotten, even more was deliberately destroyed. Except that what once existed in the minds, hearts, and bodies of the Old Ones can never truly be lost, for we are their descendants and so it is ingrained in our minds, hearts, and bodies. It remains within, waiting to be remembered again.

The Blood of a Witch is strong—stronger than many might think and stronger than some might wish—and through the generations it has come down to us. What it takes to renew that Blood is for it to be awakened to what it once was. The old Blood, so awakened, shall then be the cause of greater remembrance, both of the Old Ones, themselves, and of the ancient ways and powers that they once enjoyed. To wake the Blood is to remember who and what you once were and to remember what the Gods are, to remember what it is to be a Witch.

It is but the first step back. It is also a step forward on the path that will lead to a place that is not really a place, but all places, and a time that is not really a time, but all times. This concept has long been attached to the idea of the Witches' circle, but they more truthfully describe the *first circle*, of which all other circles are but made in the image of. As a stone cast into still water creates ripples, so all other circles ever drawn are reflections of this first circle, ripples and echoes. Each time we draw a circle, we do so in memory of that first circle, and we call upon its power.

Understandably, this first circle has had many names over the years for it spans all of time and space. It is where Witches traditionally gather, Witches of the past and Witches of the future, Witches in this world and in all others. It has been known as Benevento, Blockula, the Brocken, Mount Olympus, Venusburg, the Valley of Josephat, just to name a few and what it is, in essence, is the reality behind all the old stories of the Witches' Sabbat.

As the Witches' Mountain, it is the highest peak upon which they come together to dance and fEast and battle for the turning of the seasons and the fertility of the fields. It is the literal "world mountain," a symbol of the center of all things. But as the form it takes depends in part upon what you bring to it, what you expect and desire to see, so it may take on the appearance of not just the high peak of a mountain, but a field of roses, a castle, a great hall, or even a haunted and hidden valley.

If you truly wish to be *Sorgitza*, to be *of the Blood* as was meant by the Old Ones, then the Blood must not only wake up inside you—stirring with it the old ways of Being, Knowing, Doing, and Daring—but you must also eventually find your way to Benevento, to Blockula, to the Witches' Mountain, to the Witches' Sabbat where the Gods and the Witches and spirits yet gather to play the Game which effects this world and all others.

The Old Ones, the ancient Witches, wait for us there, as do the Witches of the future, they who are our own descendants. We stand as between two passing storms, two great waves, and so face the task of building anew the foundations, the great Towers, all that which shall uphold and herald the creation of the greatest Temple of all.

It is our task to find our way back, to reclaim what has long been lost, and lend our selves and our aid to the coming future. It is our task to renew again the worship of the Old Gods, those who have diminished in strength or even slept for a time out of having been neglected or forgotten. It is our task to aid in the leap of faith and spiritual understanding that is necessary if humankind is to evolve as a race.

As it is our task to be Shining Ones, beacons of light and hope and wisdom that carry to the Earth and to those of the Earth, the essential quality of the universe and its one ultimate source, the essence of which is Love.

What is there if there is not love?
Without love, there is nothing.
Without love, why breathe?
Why live?
It is for love's sake that the marrow burns, tears fall, songs rise in joyous abandon.
It is love that brings peace in the evening.
Love brings the stars and the morning sun.

Those who do not see or understand, their hearts are closed.
And there are only two things in your wild universe that can open a closed heart.
One is divine intervention, the bolt that you call Shaman.
Two is love.
If a closed heart doesn't open to love, leave it for the bolt of the Gods.

All is only to and for and from love.
Love is the divine which exists in all of you.

Giahna, Goddess of the Center

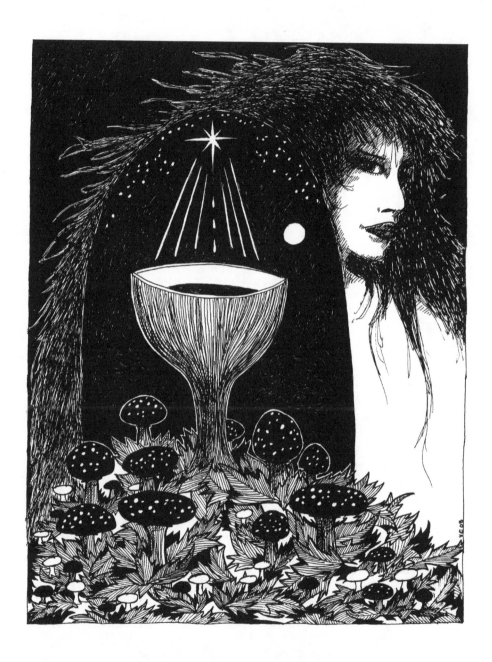

PART ONE
Witches

Long, long ago, those who would become the Witches fell to earth. They were not driven from heaven, they did not come tumbling down from grace in despair or in fear and agony most dreadful. They came out of love and they stayed out of love.

There is no greater pain and no greater gift than that.

Long, long ago, those who eventually came to be called the Witches tended to the children of man. They did so out of love and for need, for mankind was most in need of guidance.

And so great temples were raised and men learned to lift their prayers to the heavens, where the eternal stars yet reside. Not out of fear or out of despair or out of the pain of the separation from the Divine, for in those days such things were not known, but in joy for the beauty of the heavens, in happiness for the pleasures that ran in the blood and made themselves known in flesh, and in adoration of the knowledge that they themselves were made of such divinity that they could never be extinguished.

This was the lesson that those who had come from the heavens had taught. This was the lesson that the Witches had brought.

But men forgot.
And, in forgetting, took pain to their beds and fear to their hearts and so learned a darker lesson indeed.

A Legend from the Fey

The Blood

All that and more is there
As she dreams of the dance
Of rich Blood and need and fire
As she walks in her dreams
And is not afraid
Not of man nor bEast nor any God
Of earth or sky or hungry grave
Not lust, not pain, not ire
For this all she knew
And would know again
In the day, the month, the hour
When hope will turn to brave
The dawn, the wall, the moat
The twisted thorny tower
And bend to taste the breath
Of sleeping death
And remind her of her power

What are Witches anyway? Where do they come from?

Traditionally, Witches are those who are *of the Blood*. In modern times, that has come to mean those who are actual hereditary Witches. That is, those who can *prove* their Blood belongs to and descends from the ancient Witch families. Of course, this can be difficult, in part because many of us cannot trace our family history back more than just a few generations, but also because those of the Blood went underground in order to protect not just themselves, but to keep their secrets safe.

Additionally, to further muddy the waters, there have been many charlatans in recent years who have boasted of having Witch Blood and who have attempted to use that claim to further their own agendas, whether to gain power over others or to pad their bank accounts or both. However, even today, when it is far less likely that to be exposed as a Witch means a death sentence, the descendants of the Witch families of old still tend to keep to themselves, feeling little need to boast of their heritage or to promote themselves, let alone to reveal their most cherished secrets.

But, just because you cannot prove for a certainty that you may or may not have Witch Blood in your family history, that does not mean that you cannot be a Witch, for long ago those ancient Witch families interbred with those who were not of the Blood. So that today, hundreds and hundreds of years and many generations later, the Blood of the Witches of years past, has been interspersed among the general population.

It may be thin in some, weak in others, but it is there and it may be awakened under the proper circumstances. In order to wake up the Blood you must stir it up. You must rouse it from its long slumber. You have to find a way to summon the secrets that lie hidden inside it. Secrets that were put there as seeds so that they could be protected through the long years, until the time would come that they could take root and blossom forth once again. These secrets were hidden deep within the Blood so that the Witchfinders and the other enemies of Witches could not find them and attempt to destroy them, as they have tried for hundreds of years to wipe away the ways of the Blood and to destroy the last of their kind.

These sorts of secrets are the sort that can never be written down on a page and that often make little to no sense if you try to capture them that way. All that can really be written down are signposts meant to point the way to the great mysteries and magicks that are continually unfolding throughout the universe, mysteries and magicks that have powers, purposes, and personalities all of their very own. Words may aid in leading you to the proper door to those mysteries, but you still have to find the key to open that door and the courage to step through it.

Magick is itself alive. It has always been alive. So that when the magick resides in the Blood, which is also a living thing, it is doubly alive. When the spirit is invested in the Blood, in the magick, then it is triply alive. And when it comes into alignment at last with the body, with the physical vehicle through which it is meant to work in this world, then a foundation is created that can bring marvels and wonders into being.

Body, magick, Blood, and spirit, all need to come together in dynamic balance in order to make a Witch. All need to work in accord with each other in an energetic web of beauty and strength that is a reflection of how the great powers interact throughout all the worlds. For the four powers of Earth, Air, Fire, and Water are symbolic of and invested into the foundation that forms the building blocks of the universe. As they are also symbolic of our own state and of the powers that lie inside each of us, as awakened and awakening Witches, not to mention the human race as a whole.

In the past, few were invested into all four powers as a general rule— Witches followed the path of one element and so mastered that particular aspect of the greater whole. They would work together in groups then, so that each power might have representation. But, in the times ahead, it is wiser to invest in all, to learn all, and so to come into a more complete whole within yourself. Most especially since this is emblematic of the Aquarian Age which is coming into being. For when you put the four elements together, you end up with something larger and more powerful than the sum total of the parts alone.

This is also true of Witches when they create a dynamic balance between their own bodies, spirits, Blood, and the sparks of pure energy that live deep inside them. A Witch will then become, in his or her own way, a being of the Earth, of the Air, of Fire and of Water. Though, of all of them, Fire is that which relates to a Witch best, for a Witch's truest nature is of the flames and always has been. The flames that are the self-same fire that once was "stolen" from the heavens, that came down to the Earth in the form of a burning star too beautiful to bear.

But the Blood is not just something that sparks and pulses through the veins of a Witch; the Blood has a power and a purpose of its own, even a consciousness of sorts. That is to say, it is a living creature in its own right, a kind of spiritual entity. It binds Witches everywhere into one being. Each Witch is a singular spark and all the sparks come together to make up one great flame. An old metaphor for this was the way bees interacted, how they all belonged to and were connected through their hive, each contributing to build the "hive mind." It is no coincidence that bees have a long symbolic association with the Craft, a tradition that goes all the way back to the days of ancient Sumer.

Thus, to be *of the Blood* is to belong to an extended family-one whose line stretches back into the depths of history and even further than that, back to the cave of the Mothers, the cave of the beginnings, the silent place deep within the Earth when the fire first became fused with flesh and created Witchkind. But it is also to become one with a line that reaches far forward into a future as yet unknown. In this way, in the circular manner that is evocative of both natural and magickal forces, ancestors and descendants are tied together and each become as the other.

This family exists both in the lands of the living and in the realms of the dead, as well as through all of time and space. As such, a Witch is never really alone, for she or he is always in touch through the conscious power of the Blood within their flesh and bone, with all of Witchkind past, present, and future. Even though a conscious awareness of that link, of course, must be stirred to wakefulness if a Witch is to join the family in full company.

This sort of awakening usually involves passing tests of both an inner and outer nature, tests where you face down and overcome your weaknesses and claim your gifts and powers. It was exactly these kinds of tests that were once fostered and kept in the Witch families, who knew which in their generation were best suited and called to the tasks set by the Gods and by the necessities of the Craft. They knew who had the Blood and in whom it could be best awakened if needs be, who could be taught the sense of inner awareness required. They knew who had the innate ability in them to be the best at divination, at healing, at creating charms or in discovering sources of water, just to name a few examples. They knew who was called to the powers of Air or of the Earth, or to other sorts of energies, or who could be fostered in that direction if it was required.

Without their guidance, in today's age, awakenings of the Blood are far more of a mixed blessing, if you could even count it a blessing at all. Need and the Gods may call, but few may answer or even know that they should. Of those who do answer, how many more have the knowledge or ability to understand what is being asked of them, let alone are able to find teachers who have the knowledge and experience to help guide them in their blossoming role. We simply do not have the support structure in place at the present time.

21

Even worse, our current culture does not support the role of the awakening Witch in its midst—Witches being the native "shamans" of old Europe—since the Western world does not, in general, approve of native spirituality, most especially the native spirituality of its own heritage. Oddly enough, it tends to deny vehemently that Europe ever had Shamans of any sort, let alone might need their healing powers and guidance in the present day. Instead, science and modern medicine have taken its place as the primary paradigm, that and the religious structures which are essentially alien to the core nature of our ancestors.

Because we have lost our connection to our original cultural and religious heritage, people who claim to hear the voices of the Gods or of spirits or acknowledge having strange otherworldly experiences tend to make today's society nervous. More dangerous even can be the standard reaction of today's medical and psychiatric communities; those who are at the brink of awareness may find themselves being ostracized or marginalized or even medicated. Not that everyone who hears voices or has visions or metaphysical experiences may be going through the process of being called to be a Witch, necessarily, but it isn't something that is routinely screened for when one goes to see a psychologist or psychiatrist.

Another problem is that without the support and belief of the community and without the guidance of those who have experience in such matters, awakening powers and abilities may go back to sleep again if given half a chance, or go the opposite way and drive someone right to the edge of madness. Without proper training, there is always the risk that it can end in all sorts of emotional, mental, and physical issues, even in a psychotic breakdown. It can be rightly said that when one is called to be a Shaman of any kind, that you either emerge from the other side a full-fledged Shaman (or Witch), quite possibly crazy, or you may even never emerge again at all.

But how do you wake the Blood? How do you rouse the fire within the Blood? How do you take the steps that will guide you into building a circle within yourself of the elemental powers and find the path that will lead you where you need to be? Equally importantly, how do you keep from "losing it" in the process?

You need to follow the signs that point to your true self, because that is the first step on any spiritual journey. These signposts can take many forms—names, images, phrases, animal totems, spirit guides, all of them puzzle pieces of a larger whole. Essentially, it is a journey of Shamanistic exploration, a journey that will take you deep inside yourself, as much as it will lead you to a better understanding of the universe around you.

You need to take yourself apart and put yourself back together again, as more of who you were meant to be all along, leaving behind the parts that never really belonged in the first place, the parts that only really served to obscure your own truest life and light. This used to happen to Shamans of the past, when in the grips of a dream or fever, they would find themselves torn apart and put back together again, a traumatic experience that rendered them fit for their new role in society.

Not that others do not face the same process in their lives, only usually at a slower pace. Because the steps towards becoming a Witch or Shaman is in some respects the same as that of seeking to become a fulfilled human being, in that you are working to create your own best self. In this process, this quest, no one else can do it for you. They cannot fill you up with what is missing or take the steps needed for you to get where you need to go. No earthly thing can do that for you either, not money, not possessions, not sex nor drugs nor all the riches and success in the world. These are, in fact, often distractions from real fulfillment. For example, there are many who have all they ever thought to strive for—fame, family, fortune, success—only to find that they still feel empty inside, that the intense longing for *something* has not gone away. That is because none of those things matter, unless you find a way to realize yourself.

Happiness and peace and fulfillment come from a whole heart, from being able to stand in the center of your own being, knowing who you are and living who you are to the best of your ability. Then and only then, will you find the meaning you long for, the lasting joy and surety of at last belonging. Only then will you know, with an absolute sense of peace, who you are and why you are here. This is being "grounded and centered" in the truest sense of the phrase, a grounding based not so much in the Earth Herself, but being grounded in the Earth of your own being. To be centered around the light that exists within your own heart, the flame which is the doorway not just to your spirit, but to all of creation. This is the balance between spirit and flesh, between mortality and divinity, all brought into a dynamic and vital accord.

To be whole you must both *feel* and *be* all of yourself. You must know with an instinctive sense the very rush of blood through your veins, the strength of your flesh and bones, the breath and name that called you into being, as well as the fire that consumes your heart and bids you to do what you are meant to do. You will then know with a joyful surety, previously unknown, your place in the scheme of things, and how what you do and who you are affects all of life around you. As you will know that the outer world is a reflection of the inner, which are all steps down the path of an understanding, necessary to work the greatest magicks.

However, in order to speak to your soul, you must first learn how to speak to your heart. And you must listen to it, as well. For this is the first language, a language of pure knowing and one that always rings true. It is a language beyond words, a language of the spirit encased in flesh, a form of communication which understands by coming into perfect communion with what is meant to be understood.

Some old phrases that express this include the idea of having a "heart to heart" conversation or of learning something "by heart." For the head has only recently been granted the title of being the source of thought and consciousness. In years gone by, it was the heart. As to speak from the heart was to speak the truth and to see with the heart was to see the truth.

So it is that Witches need to open to their hearts, which shall tell them what is proper and meet, and what must be done by the dictates of the Gods and out of necessity. In this way, we are all travelers who have come a long way and have a long way yet to go, both to return to who we once were and to take the far road to the future. The trick of it is knowing which path to take, and to do that you must learn to listen to the voice inside you that already knows the way. You must listen not to your fears or your doubts, or even your desires, but to the voice of your spirit, the voice of who you really are.

The voice that calls you home again.

The Past

In the Ardennes, along the Danube, the Witches gathered for circles, male and female together. In the circle they exchanged their knowledge. The men knew magick and the women knew channeling energy and healing. It wasn't important for the women to learn what the men knew, just to understand it.

The men learned their magick by going to the overworld, the sky. The women learned their channeling and healing by going to the lowerworld, under the earth. This was done in separate groups, segregated by sex. The women instructed the young women. The men instructed the young men.

When they joined in circle they taught one another and they each drew down the God or Goddess respectively and came to know the divine through this contact. Not only contact with the divine itself, but through seeing it within each other.

Then they danced and danced and danced and, finally, joined…

An old story told by Ardwena, Goddess of the North

Secrets aren't just about remaining silent. Secrets are also about letting *what must be* come in its own time and in its own way, for some things are only born from silence and the keeping of silence. It does no one any good to tell them something they are not ready to hear, let alone if they are currently in a state of not being capable of really understanding. Because this kind of understanding is not of the thinking kind—something that people are pretty good with in the modern age—but something that must be learned through experience, for it comes from a far more intangible source.

This sort of innate understanding was something quite natural and normal to Witches of ancient days. It took them into direct contact with the powers that lie behind the mask of the world, powers that they could feel as they moved in conjunction with the words and actions of ritual and magick. They did not have to guess at the nature of healing plants for they could sense what virtues they would impart, a talent long since lost. They could also sense the energies that suffuse the land and tie their own work into them.

A Witches' inherent knowing does not rely on the five senses of sight, touch, smell, hearing, or taste. It is a spiritual way of knowing that relies instead upon the heart being open, forming a connection with the plant, animal, power or person that you need to understand. In this way, through the power of pure knowing, a Witch becomes almost one and the same with what she or he is focusing on and connecting to. It is an instantaneous, spontaneous almost, joyful experience that leads you not only into a more natural connection to this world, but to other worlds. A sight behind a sight, a vision beyond a vision.

In order to touch the past, we have to learn to be at one with the past, to open ourselves up to an experience of it, and through this come to an intimate understanding of just how the Old Ones thought and felt and lived. By awakening the sleeping power in the Blood we can then come to know not only ourselves, but who we were in lifetimes long ago. We can connect to those others we knew in the past, whether they are here with us again in this life or not. We can walk in the way of the Witches of old, feeling as they felt and knowing as they knew.

This is important because the Sabbats in ancient times were as much altered states of consciousness as they were celebrations tied to a particular place or season. The powers that were called upon and raised were as much within each Witch as they were in the sacred hilltops or the secluded valleys or forests where the rites took place, for we are all filled with webs of energy in much the same manner as the Earth. To work with one is to work with the other, as the inner reflects the outer and the outer reflects the inner.

In this way, when we activate those webs inside us, we also activate them in the Earth. We spin into physical being the patterns of energy brought down from the sky, the patterns of the Nameless Ones, who wear no other form than what is given to Them by purpose. In this way, Witches in their rites do not just work as pattern makers, but can become as patterns themselves; they can be masks for powers that otherwise could not walk upon the land. They are focus points and channels for living energies that are needed to renew the spiritual energy of the planet, to guide and to protect it from harm. In this process, we follow the map laid out by the stars, which is the woven tapestry of the Divine, the Compass Rose of the Gods.

To be clear, Witches of old entered altered states of being when they attended their rites and so became as one with the very patterns they created, whether old patterns or new ones. Witches were one with the body of the land and with the spirit of the land and they moved in tune with the living energies that have come to be called ley lines. They worked with the guardian spirits of the area, with the powers and forces of creation, destruction, and mutual sustenance.

The Old Ones entered a state of mind where much more is possible than is thought of today within the modern framework of science. What they could do and achieve while in that state is now dismissed as mere fancies or the delusion of an uneducated past, an invention of the superstitious minds of poor peasants. Flying in the air? Nonsense, that never happened. Gravity is an immutable law. Healing by a simple laying on of hands? Only the desperately deluded would ever trust in that. Shapeshifting? Now you really are going too far. It was mass hysteria and lack of a proper education that made people believe in such fantastical things, when everyone knows that nothing like that was possible, nor ever could be.

That does tend to be what people believe today. And belief does matter, there's no way around that. But, since how we think today is not how people thought years ago, it has made the world of the past seem almost alien to us, something we have difficulty understanding, so much so that by judging it by the current belief structure we do it a great disservice. Belief creates, belief changes things, and this results in living in a world today where flying and shapeshifting are impossible, or at the very least, highly unlikely. But it wasn't always that way.

Adherents of science and "reason" have done the Peter Pan equivalent of saying "I don't believe in faeries" and caused faeries everywhere to drop down dead. Or so they might wish to have us believe, as they would have us subscribe to the worldview that life is made up of plain black and white facts. But we can still choose to clap our hands and say with heartfelt conviction "I *do* believe in faeries" and so bring them surging back to life again. We can have a rainbow of existence, where not just one view is seen as the only correct one—the linear scientific paradigm which is already showing its limitations and blind spots, the cracks through which the greater universe can peer through.

The Witches of the past did not have a narrow worldview. They did not look at the skin of reality and go around claiming this is all there is. They knew otherwise; they didn't have to guess. They didn't think in terms of this versus that, black versus white, good versus evil. They could step in and out of other states of mind, which are worlds and realms in their own right, and perform what we might call today miracles and marvels.

Of course, one could shapeshift. Of course, one could fly. All it required was belief in a world—and so to step into such a world—where it was not only possible, but entirely routine and ordinary. You understood, with that innate sense, the animal that you wished to become and then believed yourself to be it with such complete and utter conviction that the material form took its shape from the force of the spiritual wish and essence. The same with flying. Light as thistledown? But of course, you can become one with the wind or go into a realm where gravity has no grip over you anymore. It was as easy and as difficult as that.

The Old Ones stepped in and out of worlds all the time, worlds of mind and worlds of body and worlds of spirit. They did not see them as separate as most do today. Just as they did not see time in the same way. The Old Ones were not blind to who they had been or who they would someday be. They knew without a doubt that they were of a nature as circular as the slowly turning wheel of the sky. They knew that from the center you could see all and that from there, time stretches forth around you in all directions, so you can go to any time and any place you need and desire to.

But in order to understand the world of the Old Ones now, we have to learn to think as they did then. Part of this demands that we return to an understanding of the old Witch language that they used, for within it are clues to recovering the culture and belief structure that went hand in hand with it. That is because a language is so much more than just a collection of words which have come to symbolize various objects or actions. A language is an intrinsic and necessary part of any culture, which explains it being one of the first things that a conquering race or religion will try to take away from the indigenous people. The native cultures of North America are still recovering from the losses endured by not being allowed to raise their children to use their own language and to keep their old traditions.

To lose your language is to lose an important part of your heritage, perhaps one of the most important aspects of it. Words have power and a history and within the history of those words you can find the history of a particular culture. You can find their core beliefs and their myths and legends, what holds them together as a distinct people. In this way, a native tongue is a living part of any nation as it links together not only the separate individuals who reside in it, but all the generations who pass through it.

But most languages today, including English, are sorely lacking in true communion. Our words have become too rooted in the concrete, in singular meaning. Language is meant, however, to bridge the gap between one thing and another, and so can be seen as a spell in a way, magick that is meant to negate the illusion of separation. At the same time, language has the power of creation, and a religious language even more so. Some cultures have managed to retain a "special" language for just that purpose, a language of their Gods and of their spirits and rites of worship. It was this same sort of language that the Old Ones had, that Witches once used.

Like any other language, it does involve the spoken word, but the spoken word is but the smallest part of it and not the most essential one. It is actually a more evocative language, mystical and mythopoetic in nature. For example, there is a word that means "fox," but when it is used it means not just an actual physical fox, but all that fox means in myth and legend and symbol and how all those meanings are intimately connected to each other all at the same time. As if with one word you spoke an entire paragraph, a poem even, and did not just mean one singular material thing; you feel all that fox is and ever was in that single moment.

When you speak a language that is only in part "material," then you are getting into the realm of oracles and the Gods of old. Oracles tended to speak in riddles, because riddles were the only way to bridge the gap between the greater workings of the universe and the lesser ones. For in the leap from the Divine to the material, many things must, of necessity, take the form of riddles or paradoxes, for it is difficult in any other way to express something that is beyond the "absolutes" of the physical world.

In order to comprehend these riddles, to try to see what is really meant, you must learn to think outside the box and to see past the surface of things. You must understand in the old ways, which was not really an understanding of reason, of figuring things out, but more like a light suddenly going off the dark, a leap that you can't otherwise explain. You just suddenly *knew*, and you knew that what you knew was true.

Poetry, riddle and paradox are the ways that the Divine attempts to make itself known in the more limited world we live in on a day-to-day basis. This is a language that we can enter into by coming to an understanding of what is meant by listening through the gate of the heart, which comprehends things in a different fashion than the mind does. For the heart understands the higher truths, the heart understands what is sooth.

Oddly enough, the word "sooth," which is part of the old name for those who prophesized - soothsayers - has come to mean fantasy or something made-up and so less than true or real. But the word sooth used to mean what was imparted was something higher and truer even than "truth." Truth, in the old sense of the word, was less true than sooth—for sooth was a kind of truth made known by the universe, by the Divine, by the Gods, and was that which was fated to be. Truth could alter and change, while sooth did not.

So language is important, for it keeps the inherent truths, the inherent sooth, of the culture which it is a part of. What a culture and its people share in and believe is built into its words and how those words relate to each other and to the world at large. The religion of a people is hidden in their language, expressed in their language. It is a spell of communication and of the creation of a similar worldview, a story brought to life.

In this way, all sorts of people upon the Earth are engaged in making a charm of creation. All culture and all religion proceeds from the makings of that charm, from the worlds that the spell brings into existence. For words have of old, great power and names are the forces of creation in concrete form. To change the world, you can create it anew through your belief and by an act of language tied to that belief. For a powerful enough faith and ritual can transform anything.

Still, language includes not just the spoken and the written word, but the ancient art of symbols. Symbols are, in fact, a more powerful form of language because they are a silent one, one that directly bypasses our conscious minds and goes to the depths of our selves and where we all came from. They speak to the part of us that yet remembers the cave of the Mothers from which we are descended, the Cave of the Beginnings.

The Cave of the Beginnings *is* a symbol, but it's also a deeply buried memory inside all of us. It is the "place" where Earth and Water met to form the clay made to hold the spark of life and the breath of spirit. Remembrance of this cave remains inside all things of the flesh and to go back to the beginning, back to this cave, is to seek the treasures that remain hidden there, the treasures of the fertile earth and of the deepest waters. They are wellsprings inside us, as they also form wellsprings upon Mother Earth.

It's here that any act of creation must start, because if you want to create something new, you have to go back to the beginning in order to bring it into being, especially something which has never before existed. The ideas and energies come from beyond, but to bring them into material existence they need to put on flesh, to become matter. This takes the power of the Earth and the power of the Water together to make a vessel for the breath and fire you wish to place inside them.

That creative act also requires giving something a name, for to grant a name is also part of bringing it into being. For this reason, Adam was said to have named all the animals and plants in the Garden of Eden, and for this reason those who practice the Art tend to keep their true names to themselves. For to know a thing's name is to hold power over it, the power of conjuration and the power of essence.

Conversely, if you forget who you really are, your true name and nature, then you risk going out of being. You risk becoming other than who you were meant to be by the Divine. This is not the name that you were most likely given by your parents when you were born, but the name that really signifies your spirit. It is the name that traveled with you from the Otherworld, the name that was given to you by the Divine.

To know a thing's name is to hold power over it. To know your own true name is to know your own power, to behold your rightful place in the universe. It's to be in touch with what you are supposed to be, your essential nature. When you know your essential nature, then you can strive to be that nature in all ways, and the more you are your own nature, the brighter you will shine. Like dewdrops caught in a spider's web, like the scattering of stars across the night sky, like light moving across the waters—you will be a Shining One.

Gods and angels and Faery shine so very brightly, precisely because they know who they are. They have no doubt of it for they believe and as they believe, they know. They have both faith and surety in equal measure, knowledge and belief in mutual accord. Their names are their essence and they have become their essence.

The Future

To shine with God's power, the halo of the Saints, and the crown of Kings is to stand as close to the Source inside you as you can and yet remain of the earth. It should shine through you like a prism, a pure pane of glass, a rainbow between this world and the next, between all the worlds high and low, each more beautiful than the last.

To be a shining star of your own, a glorious one, a sained one is to be made sanctified by the presence of the Divine inside you. Saints let God manifest through them—the shape of the angel or God or Goddess they will one day become...

Each mask is different. All masks are special. We are masks as much as the Gods are masks. They just know better who They are, who They have been, and who They shall be.

But why do we need to awaken the Blood? What are Witches here to do?

In regards to those of us of European descent, it's part of reclaiming our heritage, our culture, our roots. For what was lost over the past thousand or more years was not just a scattering of a few magickal spells or mystical rites, but an entire culture complete with its own language, ideals, needs, understandings, and purpose. What was lost was an understanding and purpose which infused a people with the power and knowledge to be able to help guide and heal and protect both the Earth and the human race. For Witches were, at one time, not just a few special individuals with well-developed psychic abilities or spirit contacts, but a race somewhat different from human beings.

When the Roman Catholic Church hunted down and attempted to destroy all of Europe's Witches, it was case of ancient genocide. It was an attempt to destroy the Blood and all that the Blood meant to the peoples of those lands, for the native beliefs and Witches of Europe stood in the way of the Church's wish to have complete dominion over the Earth and over the minds and hearts of all of mankind. But by that time, those of the Blood had already mingled with the human race and they could not be completely eradicated. The Blood had gone underground, so to speak, awaiting its chance to be renewed and to reveal itself once more.

That time is now upon us. The tides are changing and so the Old Ways are returning to lend their grace to a new world, to the new age rising up like a shining phoenix in the Eastern skies. The Old Gods are returning and everywhere beacons are being kindled to herald the coming dawn, bright fires that are, in themselves, signposts of a larger purpose. Witches are awakening—and must continue to awake—to the need for their existence and guidance.

It was for this that the Witches of ancient days gave their blood, so that it could be reclaimed in the future and lend its aid to the human race in making the leap into the coming age, the Age of Aquarius. For this new age heralds a necessary return to the proper respect for the interconnectedness of all things, especially that of humans and nature. Where the world will come to acknowledge the powers and abilities that science currently scoffs at, though they are the same powers and abilities that our ancestors once had and that many native cultures yet retain, even in this so-called modern age.

It also means rebuilding the communion between those of this world and those of the spirit realms. It is no coincidence that many fantasy books have as their theme the idea of the return of magick to the world or the return of Faery—they are tapping into a deeper truth that has been not only promised, but woven into the very fabric of reality. Their stories are heralding a dream and a time long foretold.

The renewal of interest in the Old Religion, the renewal of faith in the Old Gods, is also part of that return. It's an indication that the time is now for magick and mystery to come back to the world. Not that it ever really left us, for it is we who were wrapped instead in a shroud of forgetting and lost the ability to see and touch and know spirits and magick the way our ancestors did. In remembering how to do that at long last, we will also remember our selves, our past, and our power.

To wake and to remember, these are all steps that need to come first, especially so that Witches will be able to fulfill their purpose here. Because a Witch's job is not just to be here for themselves or even just for other Witches, others of the Craft; Witches are here for the Earth, which happens to include the human race. Understandably, we have a lot of work to do in the coming years, during the changeover from the old Age to the new, and on into the future

It's the work of a Witch to heal those who come to him or her, to guard the Earth, to teach, to work in keeping the powers in their proper balance, and to help guide others towards an ever greater understanding of this world, of the Otherworld, and of their own truest selves. A Witch needs to do the necessary work for the planet, the energy points, the animals and plants, and the people. Whatever aspect of the work we are drawn to fulfill.

There are lots of jobs for those called to the Craft. We all need to do the ones we came here for, that we were born for, the job we are best suited to. That goes for whether you are a Witch or not, of course. But in order to do the job properly, a Witch needs to be as whole and healthy as possible in mind, body, and spirit. This is the first step for any awakened or awakening Witch—to heal him or herself, so that they may best serve the Gods and the Earth.

One of the goals for the future is to help teach people of today how to respect both the flesh and the spirit, and how to keep the two in dynamic balance. Unlike the lessons of the past two thousand years—where the spirit was emphasized over the flesh and the flesh even called evil—we need to learn again how each reflects the other, just as this world reflects the Otherworld and the Otherworld reflects this world. How both the material and the metaphysical need and rely upon each other.

Another path that needs to be explored and shown to others is the path of joy, rather than the road of pain, loss, failure, conflict, and endless struggle. People of today know that road entirely too well, as pain and suffering has been the marching theme for most major religions for centuries. In fact, it is so deeply ingrained in our culture that we can't even begin to conceive of living in a world where it isn't true. But that is only one road among many and we have the chance and the choice to pick another to explore at this time.

A hallmark of the Piscean Age was two things pulling against each other—two fish swimming in opposite directions—and so the past two thousand years has focused on *this* versus *that*. Light versus dark, up versus down, man versus woman, good versus evil, man versus nature…the list can go on and on and we know it well already. Struggle and conflict can be a great teaching tool and the Piscean Age, like all Ages, was in fact meant to be a time of learning for the human race as a whole. But the division has also lead to a lot of pain, confusion, hatred and wars that have continued on through countless generations, as well as seeing the Earth as something to be used and exploited rather than honored and treasured.

Unfortunately, what some religions and scientific dogma has given us by adherence to this divisiveness is a belief that we have the right and authority to run roughshod over nature. It has given us a rather flat and mechanistic view of the marvelous universe all around us. Because of modern science and many mainstream religions, we have inherited a very limited world and a very restrictive worldview. Not that all of science is bad and not that there is no good to be found in mainstream religions, for there are believers and mystics of all faiths and creeds who try to honestly help others and who choose to bring light and healing into the world. So long as no faith claims that it has a lock on some One and Only Truth, it can be open to change and to acceptance of its sister faiths. In that way, the multitudes of religious paths form a rainbow—many colors that come together to make one great light, for we need the many to make the one.

There is no one, right, true, and only way. There is only the one, right, true, and only way for *you* in this lifetime…if you choose to accept the mission, that is. It's the path that you are meant by fate to walk, and even then you still have the right of choice, the right of refusal. You can turn away from your destiny or embrace it willingly; those are the options always available to anyone. Though, to walk hand in hand with Destiny, means that you will be walking in accord with your bliss and doors will open for you as never before.

Walking the path of the willing is by far the better decision, especially as the Aquarian Age is a path of wholeness and of joy. Which sounds really good, some might say, but how to we get there from here? Well, for one, people need to learn how to experience and trust in joy again, to believe in the prosperity of the universe around them. They have to figure out who they are and the meaning of their life and how to be that, as fully as possible each day. Not an easy step to take, especially here in the very beginnings of the age, but as momentum builds, it will become more and more natural, easier to learn and to express.

But what can we do to help it along? The most powerful way of teaching is not by telling someone what to do but by showing them, by being an example. It's by living the life that you hope to inspire others to live. Actions are intrinsically far more powerful in this regard, because words have a harder time inspiring lasting change unless they come at just the right time and in just the right place. So the best way to help people is by being an example yourself. In that way, simply by existing, you will be able to touch others and teach them. By just being around them, you will help all those who are open to the process to make the changes needed to become a vital part of the coming age.

Unlike most of the human race, though, Witches must consciously choose this path. Witches always choose. Hence, Witches must make the choice to ride the wave, to sail the storm, to walk with their eyes open—and with their hearts open—into the new world, the new age. A Witch is here to *do*, and so words are simply not enough. There are many kinds of magick, but Witch magick always means doing. It means taking action and causing direct transformation of the world on all levels, both Seen and Unseen.

Witches are those who know who they are. Witches are aware of what they are. Witches do what they are meant to do…by choice, not blindly. Witches choose and Witches do. So it is that Witches must, in full awareness and consciousness of their act, choose to make the leap of faith and take on the qualities of the Aquarian Age. Witches must have faith in themselves and believe and celebrate in boundless joy and love. For this is the first and best way of being a good teacher.

Witches should hold firm to the knowledge that if we but apply the powers of love and will, we can change the world for the better. For if people saw the beauty of the world, cherished it and loved it, then they would take better care of it. But, so many cannot see the beauty around them, since they cannot see it first in themselves. As they can't really love the Earth or other people honestly and truly, if they can't love themselves. But these are all steps forward, a way to walk into a future of blinding brilliance and beauty.

Men walk as though in a dream, but Witches have to be aware of the dream—so they may alter it. But the Age of Aquarius, the Age of the Star is coming and it is time for the human race to awaken to its true nature. Witches must lead the way for they know what it is that imparts awareness and can light the beacons to guide those who will follow. They can feel and hear and understand what the Blood is telling them, and know where it will lead the rest of mankind when the Blood stirs within them, as well.

Witch Blood is living blood, conscious, and this means, in part, that the Craft is much more than what most might imagine it to be. It is a living and conscious thing, a singularity made out of a multitude, so that what can actually be seen of it is just the tip of the iceberg. The greater part lies below, in the deep and secret waters, the hidden channels of power that extend across space and time. In general, we today can but barely grasp the questions of the Art, let alone make the attempt to comprehend the answers. Part of that is because we were not brought up to see past what is taught as "normal" these days and if we do, it is soon driven out of us by what Western society now believes is absolute reality.

The rites and rituals of a Witch are meant not just to work magick, but to gift the ability to see beyond masks, below the tip of that iceberg. This practice is meant to lead you to those deep waters and there to connect with ancient and powerful channels. As they are also meant to allow us to gain the vision to see the forces that flex and work and dance and sing in the Unseen realms, that which the material world overlays. This is not to say that the physical world is unimportant or that what we do and say here is of no import. For those Unseen powers can be called into account, persuaded into action, tweaked and twisted and roused by the authority of word, gesture and ritual, because the corporeal world does have an effect on the non-corporeal realms.

Though, of course, all objects, words, gestures and rituals are actually secondary tools to the intent of the Witch. This intent springs from the heart and from the will—for all right action stems from the center of being and from existing in accord with the correct functioning of the greater universe. If action and intent do not spring naturally from the heart, then they will prove ineffectual in the long run and perhaps even harmful in the short term. Because, though you can force an unnatural magickal act upon the structure of the universe, eventually the natural flow will win out.

The far better choice is to work in tune with the flow rather than against it. This brings you in accord not only with your own nature, but also with the nature of all that is. It's always a good idea to have the web of destiny working for you, rather than against you, forming a smooth and silken strand, beautiful and strong, rather than a tangle which will eventually have to be undone.

Of course, the choice is ours and always will be. A large part of being a Witch is having that power of choice. But to make the best choice, the most lasting one, it has to come from the heart, from knowing who and what you are and why you are here. Those who succumb to anger or hate or doubt or shame, who focus their life's energies in that direction or on acquiring mere *things*, have not yet found in themselves the capacity for self-understanding. They may even lack, for this lifetime, the spiritual capacity to know pure Love—what some call *agape*—which is key to being able to truly touch the Divine.

When you look around, you can see there are many people who have been badly hurt in mind, body, and even in spirit. That these people sometimes lash out against everyone around them, even those who desire to help, is no fault of their own, for they have lost touch with their own selves and are now wanderers in a greater darkness. A darkness where they will either find the light once more, or run away from it forever. This dark is not evil for it is just part of the Void, the traversing of which is a test in and of itself. But no matter how seemingly fragile the light of your own individual spark may seem, even in the darkest of times, so long as you keep tight hold of it and do not lose faith in yourself, you can and will find your way home again.

This takes courage, of course. It demands that you *seek out* your own truest self, your innermost nature, and that you do not forsake hope. For hope is nearly as great a power as love is, and hope is the golden light of the dawn which always marks new beginnings. At this particular time, it also marks the coming age, the rebirth of the Craft, and the return of Faery and of magick, as well as being a clarion call for the first faltering, yet determined steps that humankind is about to make into a much larger universe, a universe of illumination and spiritual unity.

All it takes is to open your heart and to learn to see with the eyes of the heart. This is what the Craft must seek to give those who walk its hidden worlds, who desire to light the path to show the way for others who come after. Because, to focus on fear is to usher in fear and to concentrate on pain and loss and anger is to give them power over you and over this world. It risks opening the door to yet another Dark Age, rather than one of light. It's a choice we all have to make, whether to wither away or to accept the challenge and go forward into the future to make it live and thrive anew.

What is Witch Blood? As the Gods tell us, *"the Blood is in everyone—some know it, some do not. Some refuse the knowledge of it. It must be awakened. Some refuse to be open to it. The Blood can be awakened in anyone open to it."*

Covens

We held hands.
We formed a circle, a circle within a circle.
We were as we always were and yet not. We did not yet know who we had been, nor what we could yet attain to.

We stood together, on the edge of the Abyss.

That's where it always starts.

A single shared sound rises from many voices, creating a voice combined. We are those voices. We are that voice. A coven is made up of many voices bonded together for one shared purpose, one shared path. Of course, you might not necessarily know all the time where that path might lead you or what might end up being asked of you as an individual or as a group. In the end, the most you can do is to walk that path to the best of your ability and put your trust in the rest.

When in a coven, as in the wider world, each of us holds a different strand of the thread, but none can entirely see the wider weave we are creating together. We are all weavers, of course, but we are also part of the web, which can make it hard at times to see past just that piece we hold in our own two hands. But yet that same web, that great tapestry, exists inside us all and has its reflection within our hearts and can be found there, if nowhere else. Because this pattern is part of all we know and exists both all around us and inside us at the same time.

To be in a coven in some ways can be like traveling with a bunch of people to an event you all want to attend but have never been to before. You can see the road right in front of you, you can see the road right behind you, but the destination lies out of sight, except for a few signposts you might pass along the way. Because we are on this journey together, though, we can pool our resources, which means that going as a group can sometimes take you farther than going it alone. When you are all committed not just to each other but to a common goal, you can share your skills and knowledge and experiences with each other and be an encouragement and source of strength if someone falters along the way.

Still, though a coven can be there for you, you have to master each test along the way yourself, because no one else can give you the inner strength, insight, and resolve to withstand the hardships and the difficulties that you and you alone need to overcome. If they did, then you wouldn't really learn and you wouldn't really be on a journey. Because spiritual journeys are all about the going, not about the actual getting there. This is something that gets forgotten on occasion, especially in a very competition driven society.

It may sound like a wicked twist of fate, but if you don't learn what you need to learn along the way, then you won't be able to see what you were looking for when you finally get there. It might be right in front of you, large as life, but you won't be able to see it, because you aren't really ready to; you missed out on acquiring the necessary tools and insights that should have come with the journey. It's like a game in that way, one where you have to find a key hidden somewhere in a maze before you can open the door to the castle that lies at the far end, a maze filled with sWitchbacks and misleading turns, as well as dragons and other obstacles.

We all have to pass our own tests then, but yet we can travel together on similar roads at the same time. Your companions can lessen the pain a little, especially when it really needs lessening. They can point things out that you may have been in danger of missing. They can be a sounding board for your thoughts, your ideas, your insights and even your doubts and fears. On occasion, they may even spot the edge of the cliff right in front of you, the one that you couldn't quite see, or the dragon waiting to leap on you around the next turn of the maze. Because we all have our "blind spots" and there are always times when we hesitate, unsure of ourselves and of what we might be getting into. Learning to trust others is as much a test as learning to trust in ourselves.

Magicians of old walked a far more lonely path than Witches ever did, a fact that even the Inquisition knew. Which is not to say that you cannot be a Witch alone, but that once you have experienced a coven of shared purpose, a coven where each spark lends itself to the central flame, a coven that *is* a star-filled crown upon the earth…then you will also feel the living power of magick as it spirals and rises up from the bodies of the coven. You will sense your own spirit lifting and joining with the rest, and know the beauty of being one in the many and many in the one. You will be a Witch that is part of the greater family.

So we come to dance together as *Sorgitzak*, Witches all, each one of us with a raised candle in our hand. We weave the threads of our own selves into a magickal tapestry of souls. We spin and dance and turn, reflecting the soul of a coven that is made in the image of a wheel, one that spins and dances and turns around a central point, and so spins out the seasons, the years, and even the Ages. As voices rise together into their own web, making a song of being, of creation, of change, of prosperity and plenty, whatever is most needed for this particular time and place.

For a coven is *communion*, above all else. It is formed of shared breath, shared life, shared purpose and resolve. When a coven is united as one, you can see yourself in the eyes that look back at you, as they can see themselves in your own eyes. The same way that we look at the Gods and They look at us. For we walk the path together with Them, as well. We trust in Those who have set our feet to it and ask that we walk, even if we and They might not always know where the path will take us.

Of course, people join covens for many different reasons. Some come seeking knowledge and power. Others come for a sense of family, to find that which they had not known with those they had been born to. Many come to learn of the ways of worship, to form relationships with the Old Gods. While others come to work magick and do healings, or to discover the Divine deep within themselves.

From all directions they come and to all directions they go and every person brings a new perspective and new gifts, new hopes and dreams. Which is as it should be, for a coven is a braided rope, a single strong line made up of many threads. Not that everyone knows right away exactly why they are there, nor how they will fit in, but if they listen to their hearts and to their teachers—whether they be the Priestess or Priest of the coven, or to the Gods Themselves—then they will find signs and omens and portents to help guide them along the way.

In this manner, a coven is not so much a teaching tool as a gateway to being. Each Witch joins and forms part of the whole, which is Witchcraft. A Witch alone can find it twice as hard to get half as far as one who joins a coven which is united in a pure and like purpose and chooses to walk their conjoined path with honor, faith, and passion. A coven is a group which binds each member's singular energies into one resolve. A proper coven may not just whisper together, but dance, sing, and raise up the elemental powers of the universe together, focusing them on their proper usage.

When a coven works as it should it *is* magick, pure and undeniable. This happens when those who are a part of it strive to be the best they can be and to work together in harmony to face the challenges that they are given. Of course, some people talk the good talk, but then refuse for whatever reason to walk the good walk. Words can only count for just so much, since some people are great liars, especially those who lie to themselves. While, others mean well, but fail to follow through. When it comes down to it, what you really have to pay attention to is what people *do* far more than what they *say*. This way you can honestly judge the worth of someone, be they a coven mate or even your Priest or Priestess.

Actions are the telling mark of who a person really is and how they view the world deep down inside. Setting aside the picture that they have painted with their words, no matter how pretty or smart or how convincing, what is it that their actual deeds, or misdeeds, are telling you? Do they actually practice what they preach, or is it only a mirror that they hold up to others in order to find them wanting?

The same goes for a coven and the actions a coven takes. Does a coven walk the path it claims to walk? Does it make good use of the gifts that each Witch brings to it, or does it ignore some, shut others out, and generally become a tool for those who are running it? Because joining a coven is about getting connected. You become a part of something that is larger than yourself. Something that is larger even than those who are your teachers and who you attend ritual with. You become a part of something that has a life of its own, even a consciousness, one that you lend your life, time, and energies to. So it is especially important to be sure of what purpose those energies are being put to, because you will bear responsibility for it.

You become tied to those Witches who form your coven, especially when you do a lot of magick and ritual with them. You form a greater whole with them. For if each person is a star, then a coven is a constellation. It makes a picture and it has its own mythology. It spins around the center point of the heavens, the symbol of which is the North Star, the way of adventure, the high road to the Gods. The North Star then, in any coven, is not a person per se, not even one of your teachers, but the goal and purpose of the coven. It's what holds it all together and inspires it to the highest aspiration.

But the North Star—indeed, all the stars in the heavens—aren't just out there, out of reach, because they are inside us in their own way. To become connected to yourself is in some respects the same as being connected to a coven, because it will lead you to realize that what is *out there* is only a reflection of what is already inside yourself. That the central point within you is also the mystical North Star and that your life is itself a constellation of stars, one that forms a story, a mythology, a pattern.

When you follow your pattern, your mythology, you revel in what you are most meant to be and shine all the brighter for it. You become part of a ring of stars, one that with each star that is added, the light that is sent out into the world is magnified a thousand fold. So each coven of Witches is more than the sum of its parts, more than those who stand hand in hand within the circle that they have created, their physical bodies wick and wax to feed the flame rising within their hearts. An awakened Witch can claim that he or she is of the Clan of the Stars, whose family of the heart is of the Gods Themselves, and whose blood is linked to the royal blood of those who first walked upon the Earth.

This, then, is a coven in its first, best incarnation—a being of shared wine, breath, and need. A spirit of shared purpose, delight, hardship, and understanding. Witches' power finds strength in union and reflects the nature of the universe at the same time. The reason why a coven is thirteen is thus one of the riddles of the moon, something fashioned of thirteen separate faces and yet a completion at the same time.

But how do you fit into a coven? How do you know when one is right for you?

We turn to the North, to the Earth and call her, Mother. We turn to the East, to the Air, and call her sister. We turn to the South, to the Fire, and call him brother. We turn to the West, to the Water, and call him Father. We are related to all, and so through our bonds of kinship we may call upon the elemental powers of Earth, Air, Fire, and Water. These four powers are the building blocks of the universe. We have to learn to connect to them in as intimate a way as possible in order to understand them and to call upon them when the need arises.

The first order of a coven must be to build their foundation, one based upon the powers of the elements, so that you have a strong place to start from. You will need a foundation and a name, one which is tied into the purpose of your coven. Each Witch in a coven can embody a virtue of the elements, thus creating the foundation for the whole. Part of exploring our own inner natures then is to find out just what we are bringing to the family table, to the future of the coven.

The coven that is right for you is the one that speaks to your inmost self and does not shirk its responsibilities, nor shy away from the mill that grinds the grain to gold, the growing pains that we all must face in order to change. The right coven for you is the one that will take you where you need to go, even if it's only to the first bend on the road. Except that, sometimes, you will *know* not only that you have been with and journeyed with these souls before, but find yourself slipping easily into sync with them in this lifetime.

Once upon a time, covens were named for where they were located. This made sense, since they were tied to the land and invested in the local community, which was also tied to the land. When their land prospered, they prospered and in this way the coven worked for both the land and the community. But most covens today are not named for a place and do not, in general, think first of the fertility of the land in their magicks. Despite this, covens can still become a focal point for the natural energies of the area, which lend power to the magick that they do. These energies have been called ley lines, among other things.

But what is the purpose of a coven today if not specifically for the land and its fertility?

One purpose is to be of service to the community and to teach that community how to return to a proper connection to the land, for there needs to be a natural give and take, one that is respectful of both. People in the community also need guidance and healing, both for themselves and for being able to walk their own path of understanding—understanding which will lead them to see how interconnected we all are. Energies flow through cities and cultures as much as they do through the veins of the Earth, and can be turned to creation or destruction, to selfish or to honest use. They also can become bottled up and spread disease, whether physical disease or diseases of the spirit.

Witches need to insure that free flow continues, that we live with the Earth, as a part of the Earth, and not imagine ourselves separate or better than those living creatures we share it with. Witches need to be teachers and healers, spiritual counselors and living examples of the best possible future of humankind. Covens need to be tools as well as crowns of beauty and desire, living tools that are invested in life and in the vitality of growth and change.

This is a fertility of the spirit, one that fosters creativity and good will, that brings fortunate powers into alignment. There may be a call in the future for Witches to, once again, work magick for the wealth and bounty of the Earth, for what is needed to keep people fed, but there is also a great necessity in these days to rouse a community's sense of togetherness and to feed their increasingly unsatisfied spiritual hunger.

Shadows, candlelight, between the hours of dusk and dawn we hold hands as the power we raise together sweeps and whirls among us. A coven is not just a group of Witches, but a thing unto itself—a magickal creation formed from the currents of power lent it by each individual Witch. And as the coven changes—as people join, people leave, people transform—the larger being that they create also changes, it learns and grows and transforms like any other living being.

Thus, a coven name should embody the consciousness of each coven, its purpose, what form all that energy will take. To know a things' name is to have power over it, to bring it into being, so to pick a name for your self, a Craft name, is always an important choice. Equally then, the same is true in picking a coven name. This is the expression and form your group's energy will take in the inner and outer worlds, what you strive for and what drives your forward.

This makes it even more vital that what you do choose as name, whether it be for your own use or for the use by a coven, is chosen wisely and well.

male and female together

So the sun and the moon conspired
To light the world
In alternate directions,
As a man and a woman each must stare
Into the other's eyes
To find the path untaken,
To know the unknown
Element within themselves,
The key to desire.
As the dead are called to the living
And as the living reach out
To the dead,
A communion of opposites
Contained in a kiss of dread
Beauty and of fire

A lot of emphasis has been placed on the Goddess in recent years and to a return of focus on the feminine aspect of the Divine. This has been a much needed change, the unfolding of which has allowed women to once more find their own place and power in the world, including the spiritual world. However, unfortunately, this sometimes has taken place at the cost of the masculine aspect of the Divine and of the old Pagan Gods.

This imbalance, and it is an imbalance, would be in the long run as unnatural and detrimental to the Earth and the human race as an overemphasis on the masculine has proved to be. Balance means just that—balance—a dynamic and energetic polarity which emphasizes both the masculine and feminine powers in equal measure and uses their interplay in magickal work. Both Gods and Goddesses are needed, as are Priests and Priestesses, for together they form a real and metaphoric whole.

This is reflective of the universe, for all great powers are dual in aspect. This dual nature is usually expressed in pairs of "opposites," such as dark/light, night/day, up/down, male/female, life/death and, of course, good/bad. In the Age passing away, these pairs were set against each other, in particular the good/bad one. The emphasis was placed on their differences and not on how they might come together to form a unified whole greater than the sum of their two parts.

Quite often, one aspect was suppressed or defamed in order to concentrate on the other more "positive" or "good" element. In this manner, the Pagan Gods and Goddesses were either suppressed or defamed, and with them Their followers. The Old Gods were called evil or devils and when They couldn't completely be wiped out of the minds and hearts of the people, They were given what amounts to a make-over. They were turned into various Saints, their old days of celebration were given a Christian overtone, and churches were built on the bones of the ancient sacred sites.

This was done because the Christian paradigm at the time—and in some ways, still is—that of the Piscean Age. If you were not a believer in their God, who was the one right true and only God, then you could only be worshipping the devil. You had to be either on the side of good or on the side of evil. Shades of gray simply did not exist, and neither did the idea that one path may work for one person and yet not for someone else and that both were quite capable of achieving a Divine connection.

The Aquarian Age now coming into play has a rather different focus. It is far more concerned with the whole and on the creative and dynamic interplay between what might be perceived as "opposites." For these pairs not only spark off each other, they need each other. They are both repelled and drawn towards each other at the same time. They are opposed, yet reflective of each other, thus displaying in their interaction some of the cardinal rules of magick.

Working together, pairs of opposites make a song, a story, a work of art, a magickal spell of love, need, desire, and creation. They both reflect the singular nature of the Divine and its multifaceted one. Of course we, as beings of a limited physical nature, cannot comprehend the grand totality of that singular nature except in smallish doses and so it must be broken down for us. The grand Divine spins itself out into pieces, pieces that take on the aspect of a duality born of time. Gods and Goddesses and spirits…like our own selves, they take on an essence, an illusion of having a separate nature. An illusion that is also a reality, the same as a mask can be a mask, yet entirely real at the same time.

To get back to the ultimate, to explore the deeper mysteries, requires that the two conjoin as one. Which is why one symbol of that is found in the intimacy of male and female, Priest and Priestess, God and Goddess. The path of the Goddess alone is but one way and will only go so far before the nature of the Divine insists that a God aspect be served and honored, as well. If both are not acknowledged, then imbalance is the end result, whether that imbalance is skewed more to the male or to the female end of the spectrum. You are only getting half of the picture that way.

So, each of the four Quarters has its "male" and its "female" aspect, its God and Goddess face. Both are necessary to make up the totality of the Quarter. Both reflect, renew, and require each other. To the South, for example, the God is Tzahranos and He is action, will, and Doing. While, the Goddess of the South is Sahlonshai, and She is the physical element of Fire. Yet both Fire and Doing are intimately interrelated and, together, they create the power of the South.

The same is true for the Quarters of the East, West, and North. The "female" aspect, the Goddess, is related to the material or physical manifestation of the Quarter and the "male" aspect, the God, to the energy of the Quarter, the more Unseen manifestation. There is a Goddess then for the elements of Earth, Air, Fire, and Water, and a God for the elements of Being, Knowing, Doing, and Daring.

The opposite is true for the Cross-Quarters. For the South-East, South-West, North-West, and North-East, the "male" aspect is the physical expression and the "female" aspect is the immaterial energy. These aspects also have Gods and Goddesses attached to them, Gods and Goddesses whose powers are intimately related to and partake of each other.

In this way, a Priest and a Priestess may also each represent a differing aspect of the Divine, and when they work together they form a greater whole than the sum of the two parts. The ancient Witches, the *Sorgitza*, made use of this metaphor and the magickal power inherent in the idea of reflecting the structure of the Divine. They worked with the masks of the Divine as the living beings they are, yet also saw behind the masks at the same time. They were aware of the layers that make up the universe, of which only one part is the material world that we all know and live in today.

When one speaks of the Quarters, you are acknowledging two sorts of powers that are yet one power. Both powers have a consciousness that manifests as a God or as a Goddess. And when the two come together, then another consciousness is born, that of the Quarter itself, a consciousness that also has a mask and a name. It is formed of a many that is at the same time, a one.

Accordingly, each Quarter has many levels to it, each with its "male" and "female" aspect, its split reflection. There are also two kinds of spirits or beings at each Quarter, one attached to the God of that Quarter and one belonging to the Goddess. So it is that the spirits of Air are of Her, of the East Goddess, and the spirits of knowing are of Him, the God of the East. While the spirits of Water are of the Goddess of the West and the spirits of Daring are of the Western God.

Which is not to say that male/male and female/female relations cannot raise energy and do not form a magickal bond. It is simply that it is a different metaphor, a different symbol, than the one used by the *Sorgitza*. The Witches of the Old Forest used the power inherent in the dynamic interplay of opposites, whether that took the form of male and female or of light and dark or of life and death, just to name a few aspects.

When you set these opposites into place and let them work their magick, then you discover the greater singular power that lies beyond them. But, being that we live in a world of opposites, a world of time and space, we find it hard to perceive that singularity, let alone prove capable of dealing with it on a regular basis in our daily lives. It is simply too much. So that power splits into two, and from there into four, and so on. As it goes outward from the central single point, it expands into more and more aspects of itself. Aspects that naturally form themselves into pairs of opposites.

During the Piscean Age, the relationship of these opposites was to set them into conflict with each other or to deny one in favor of the other. This was done to serve as a lesson, a lesson that had to do with the nature of power. That time is now ending, so the next lesson will be to unify those opposites into an expression of the whole, or into as much an expression of the whole as is possible upon the material plane.

One way to do this is to use the metaphor of male and female, of the God and the Goddess. Not to place one over the other, or to deny one in favor of the other—both of which are Piscean traits and not Aquarian—but to concentrate upon the relationship between the two, through which you can catch a glimpse of their own initial source, which is our source, as well.

The same is true of the relationship between this world and the Otherworld, between the land of the living and the realm of the dead. We need to learn to use that reflection and not give prominence of one over the other, let alone say that one doesn't even exist. When we deny the Otherworld, we also deny this world and it loses part of its soul. Just as when we claim that nature has no rights over us, but only we over it, we create an imbalance, one that nature is suffering for and that we will also suffer for eventually, unless that imbalance is corrected. Not to forget that, when we deny the physical—another big part of the age passing away and many of the religions born of that age—we end up negating the spiritual, as well.

It's not an easy task, to find and maintain a good balance, especially after having been raised not to even believe in one. We get so used to being out of whack, to living our lives out of balance, that we begin to think this is just how the world is. That this is how it works and it can't ever change. So many people today hurt inside and can't figure out how to stop the pain. They are out of alignment with their own lives and selves and the society as it is now generally cannot or will not help them. It's just not set up to do that. Instead, distraction and medication have become the be all and end all, the solution to the vast majority of life's ills.

But if you start with the small things, with the small pieces of your life, and work your way upwards, then bigger and bigger pieces will begin to click into their proper place, their proper alignment. That's the nature of things; if you start to set your life in balance, even by only beginning with one aspect, it sends out a signal that you are seeking to work on your life here, that you are willing to change and to learn. A signal that the Gods, the spirits, and the universe at large will respond to.

The Witches' Mountain

A field of roses.
Once blood was let here,
In battle for the seasons.
Each took their side
And played the game as best they could.
White and black pawns,
Dreaming of rich crops and fertile women.
In the manor they would fEast,
And time and tide knew them not.
The heart of the maze took its chances,
Hedge Witches all,
Up the chimney and across field and flood and wind
And valley deep with shadow,
They flew to battle.
They flew to fEast.
Black and white squares surround the castle.
The chalice lies within.
The dreams poured out.
Rose petals and apple blossoms,
Spring comes.

In Germany it was called Venusburg or the Brocken—the highest and most haunted peak in the Hartz Mountain rage. In the Netherlands, they named it Blockula. In Italy, Benevento. In Fruili, they called it the Field or the Valley of Josephat. In the ancient lands of Kemet, the country known today as Egypt, it was the place now called The Valley of the Kings. The Elysian Fields. The Plain of Aphrodite. Mount Olympus. Mount Athos. The summit of the Himalayas. The depths of Kilauau. Harney Peak, the sleeping bear-shaped hill that marks the Eastern edge of the sacred Black Hills of South Dakota. Even Roswell, which means "field of roses." It has had many, many names throughout time, some of them long lost to forgetfulness, if not deliberately erased by those who would wish it never to have been.

It can take as many forms as it has names. It can appear as a mist shrouded valley, one filled with flowers, usually roses, or merely imbued with the mystical scent of blossoms. It could seem a great manor house with a fEasting hall inside, one filled with warm cheer, with every food or drink that you could desire. It could be a meadow of tall grasses with a nearby well or spring, one watched over by a lovely woman described variously as a maiden, an abbess, a goddess, the Queen of the Moon, the Queen of Faery, the Queen of the Sabbat. Or it could appear as the highest mountain peak in the region, majestic and terrifying, near enough it seemed to reach out and touch the sky.

But, whatever the name, whatever the shape, it's the meeting point of Witches everywhere, those scattered throughout all of space and time. It is where the four roads lead to and where they meet at long last to make the old "Witches crossroads." It's from this meeting place that we get the idea of a circle taking place in a place that is not a place and a time that is not a time, because *the first circle* exists everywhere and nowhere at the same time. It's both a physical place and not a physical place, also at the same time. As it spans all of time, all of history, the pivot point upon which the world and the Ages spin.

Benevento is both out of time and yet touching all of time, for it exists between worlds, both part of and none of them all. When you go there you go in spirit and yet when you go there you go in the flesh. Confusing as that may sound, this sort of paradox is part of the true Witch's Sabbat. It's part of the altered state of consciousness, of how you see the universe, required to both get there and to play the Game.

Certainly, this paradox proved confusing to the enemies of Witches hundreds of years ago, as the whole concept yet remains an intriguing enigma to today's scholars and historians of the Witchcraft craze of the Middle Ages. Was it real or not real? Did Witches attend the Sabbat physically or did they but go in spirit or even in just their imaginations? Was it ever a physical place or was it always just a mental fantasy, one perhaps brought on by the ingestion of various sorts of herbs, mushrooms, or drugs.

The answer to the essential question of whether or not the Witches' Sabbat was real is yes. As to whether it was physically real or spiritually real the answer is also yes. Both are right. Did Witches attend in the flesh? Yes. Did they attend in the spirit? Yes. While, as to the question of exotic herbs, mushrooms, or drugs...there were always ways to aid in opening the door within the mind, the doors to perceptions beyond the five simple senses. If you knew how to open that door without such aids, then you did not need them. And if you needed them to show you the way, after a time you put them aside when you could get there without their help any longer.

Call it what you will, this is the Witch's true circle, the one that every other circle in this world is just a shadow and a reflection of. For while here in the physical plane we raise circles as we are taught, the Witch's Sabbat circle, the *first circle*, is created not by those who exist in the flesh, but by the spirits of the Air, the Elder children, those who came before us. The circle that they create then has its echo in every circle drawn upon the wide earth below. It's the pattern of which all others are a shadow, by which they take their shape.

Because of the nature of such a place, in order to get to Benevento, to the Witch's Mountain, it takes many steps. The first step requires stirring up the Blood and bringing it to a wakeful state. This is done by *Dancing the Blood*, for through ecstatic dance the Blood awakens to what it is and we remember along with it. However, this needs to be done for a good while because the way has long been lost and we are ingrained with many walls and doubts that will need to be overcome in order to succeed.

The state that is necessary to achieve Benevento is, unsurprisingly, also somewhat paradoxical in nature. You must feel oddly both terribly exhilarated, almost giddy, and yet find yourself, at the same time, feeling barely able to stay awake. This is the prelude to entering an altered state of consciousness that will allow you to "fly." It is an intoxication of the spirit and not of the body, one that lets your spirit slip free of its moorings in this world.

Witches were often accused of "flying" to their Sabbat, but the sort of flying that was meant was not a literal soaring across the sky on the back of some old broomstick, but flying in the Shamanistic sense of the word. You traveled in spirit, leaving your body behind. Yet, you could also go where you wanted to go in spirit and then bring your body along after. Need and circumstance dictated the choice, as did the skills of the Witch in question.

Once a Witch attained Benevento, it was there that they sang, danced, and made merry with one another, with those they had known in the past and would know in the future. But what also takes place at Benevento or Venusburg is the Game. It's also been called "the good game" or "the game of Benevento." It may include a battle between two sides, a fight where each side represents some greater power or force—a battle which is both serious and silly at the same time—and the effects of which ripples out across many worlds. Sometimes these battles took place astride a representative of your totem animal—a dog, a cat, a wolf, a bear, an eagle, whatever represented your personal power.

For a totem animal is related to the Witch they carry and so shares certain aspects of character, both good and bad. For example, a Witch whose totem animal is a lion might have the strength of a lion, but also the feral nature and social needs of one, as well. While, someone whose totem is a magpie might find themselves good at finding things, but also end up living in a cluttered home, one filled to the rafters with all the pretty things that have caught their eye over the years.

Not that totems need to be animals or birds, because they also can be flowers or even other symbols that have magickal significance. Either way, a Witch does not choose his or her totem; the totem always chooses the Witch. It is part of the inheritance of the Blood. Just because you may adore dolphins or cats or wolves does not mean that they can be or are your totem. When your totem picks you, sometimes you do have an inkling that they might be the right one beforehand, but often as not it comes as a bit of a surprise. Only later, after you take the time to delve into the creature or thing which has chosen you as its own—when you do research and develop your own personal relationship with it—might you discover how very right it was all along.

Of course, certain animals have a long tradition of association with Witches. In particular, cats, owls, hares, pigs, ravens, snakes, toads, and spiders spring to mind. It is no coincidence that many of these are also associated with some of the old Pagan Gods. This, of course, also holds true for the Gods of the *Sorgitza*, some of whom have various animals as

Their symbols. As with the connection made to a Witch, the connection between a God and an animal lies in its representation of the aspect and flavor of the power that they symbolize. So it is, that when a Witch is called to fight during the Good Game, that he or she rides to the battle upon the back of that same power.

But what is the Game? What is it for?

We're used to thinking of games as things done simply to pass the time, to provide fun and amusement. Children are allowed to play games, while adults must justify the art, because it takes us away from more important things. We're all grown up now so we have to put away childish things, including the right to play silly, even simple games. Instead, work is stressed as being more important, though perhaps the operative word there shouldn't be work so much these days as *stress*.

But games, certainly the older sorts of games, are patterns and patterns are a part of rituals for a reason. Just as patterns are a part of natural cycles. Patterns have power. Patterns create. They build things within the structure of the mind, the body, the soul, and the universe. In a way of speaking, they create habits and these habits can be shortcuts. Why spend twenty minutes getting into the proper frame of mind for a ritual if, after many years of pattern-building, the simple usage of a couple of key words and the smell of just the right incense may do as well. But you have to put your time into the creation of those patterns first, before you abandon any aspect of them.

We have to write a pattern into our very bodies, minds, and spirits in order to be able to move beyond them. Because of this, patterns that seem almost instinctual or rhythmic, that speak to us in the language of play, mirth, fun, and imagination are the best kinds of patterns, the same as those which thrill us, which make us shiver a little inside. They take us out of ourselves as much as they allow us to go deep within and renew in us a sense of wild abandon and wonder in the world we live in.

When you learn to play the Game, only then will you be able to learn to go beyond the Game, to fathom what unseen forces move behind the mask of what you see and do. To be able to see the effects you have had in playing the Game and how it ripples across countless worlds, both the ones you are familiar with and those you are not. Worlds that interlock with and also affect each other, as your actions have effected them. You will be able to see all of this, to be a part of it and yet separate at the same moment, and know the invisible cogs and wheels, the winds and storms and currents which lie behind the movements of the material plane.

However, this is not a decision that is up any of us to make. You cannot wake up some morning and decide that you have moved past the need for patterns, that you have outgrown the structure of the game, of the ritual, and just choose to walk away from it. No, you will know when you have moved past the need for ritual when you begin not just to "see" what lies behind the patterns, but when you can "experience" them. When you can clearly sense the great web of interconnection between all things.

The feeling of this sense is unmistakable and incredibly difficult—if not impossible—to describe, at least in most languages we are left to use today. It is akin to trying to describe the depths of profound joy to someone who has never truly experienced it, or the misty splendor of a rainbow to someone who has never seen one. Words are clumsy tools to describe feelings and emotions and spirituality as it is, let alone moments that may be imagined as "peak experiences."

To go beyond the habits and patterns of the Game, or of life itself, is to step into a world where the material is but one piece of a greater whole. It's to peer into a world that operates by certain rules, some that our own mimic, and some that seemingly make no sense by what modern science theorizes to be immutable laws of nature and the universe. Though some scientific seekers are beginning to understand there is a whole lot more going on than they can explain, at least at this time.

What they seek to understand in a way is that the patterns we make do have power, not just over we who make them, but over the Unseen realms that lie all around us, that co-exist with our own world. Worlds within worlds, patterns within patterns, wheels within wheels…the universe is multi-layered, conscious, and interactive, even though we tend to see but the smallest part of it for the most part. So we play games, but what we really do is make patterns and these patterns play bigger games and make bigger patterns. We are all players and pawns at the same time.

There are many games, some large and some small, some simple and some complex. But as the greater reflects the smaller and the smaller, the greater, so no game played with purpose and intent is without its effect in the wider structure of reality. What we do in ritual is a "game," and when this gets you to the Game of Benevento, then you have achieved a larger playing field, one even closer to the hidden powers that lie behind the scenes.

But you have to participate. You have to play the Game fully, believe in it fully, in order to play it properly. However, the difficulty is, at the same time you have to not forget that it *is* but a game, or you take the risk getting caught in your own spell, in getting lost in the very pattern you are weaving. It's the same as working magick—when you are in the midst of doing the spell, you must believe in it utterly, with absolute certainty and faith that it shall work and come to fruition, even if once you step out of the ritual atmosphere you might entertain doubts.

You must believe in the Game utterly as you play it, but yet never forget that it is a game. This may seem a contradiction, but thinking in a paradoxical fashion is part of what Witches of the old ways were practiced in, for it was the key to many magicks. Reality and the world was a much more fluid thing in those days, because people believed differently than they do today; they believed that more was possible, and so it was.

There are games and games, just as there are patterns and patterns. The Witches' pattern is set here upon the Earth, but yet it is a pattern born of the night sky, of the dance of the stars. A Witches' circle is of two worlds, which makes it a reflection of the nature of each Witch, who also walks in two worlds. Worlds that find their reflection in each other, and which together give way to a greater reality.

We learn the patterns of our rites, burning them into our very minds, bodies, and spirits, so that they will lead us to the door that opens upon the patterns that lie beyond. Each pattern that is learned leads to the next. To come to see past one mask finds another staring back at you, each one more beautiful and terrible than the last. Until, eventually, you come to the most beautiful and terrible one of all, that of the ultimate. A mask which is not a mask and a face which is not a face, the same as the game which is not a game…for what is the living paradox if not the way to catch a glimpse of the Divine?

Joy and Terror

Witches must remember
Witches must return
Rise again to show the way
To those who once they spurned
Witches live in three worlds
Witches walk in two
A five pointed star to guide them
Seven points renew
Eleven dance upon the hills
And thirteen in the dark
Call to raise the power
Sing to raise the spark
Turn and turn and turn once more
And step freely through the door
To walk the mirrored hallway
They're waiting for you there
Born of fire and born of light
They hold the secret seed
Offered in a drink of blood
And wine and need.

There are two ways that the Blood may come alive and the doors open wide—the path of joy and the path of terror. Both extremes of joy and of terror sweep through the mind and body, rousing your senses, including those of the Otherworld. This is partly because they stir us to wakefulness, including a wakefulness of the Blood. It is through an arousal of self that you learn to see with infinite clarity who and what you truly are. It's how you understand what you are required to understand if you want to be a Witch and regain the Witch powers of old, powers that were an intrinsic part of them and of their Blood.

But why joy? Why terror? Terrible joy and joyful terror are feelings so strong, so intense, that they can drive you right to the edge of madness and beyond. They are ways to open doors, doors to that which otherwise cannot easily be reached. In this, both joy and terror are like opposite sides of the same coin, a coin meant to purchase your passage to worlds of fear and fascination.

Terror and joy are woven together at their core, so that you cannot really feel one without feeling the other. They share a similar nature in the way that what is absolutely beautiful is also terrible to behold, mainly because of the pain of awe that it creates inside us. We see something so beautiful that it hurts, emotionally and physically, or we are shaken by something so dire that we become, in that moment, acutely alive and aware. We become aware not just of the things of this world, but of other things, of other forces.

In this fashion, joy and terror can form a gate and open the way to inner understandings and to the mystery of the realms of the spirits. Realms which suffuse the physical world we all live in, as the spark of life suffuses our own flesh. They open our eyes to that which is always there, always around us, but yet not seen until that time, until the sight is gained. This gate balances on the fine edge of mingled joy and terror, a narrow bridge that Witches must traverse in order to learn to stand with one foot in the land of the dead and one foot in the world of the living.

Those who become aware of the spirit which resides within them may then call it forth and send it winging to other realms, to other lands and other worlds. To become aware of the spirit is to become aware of the light within, the light which comes from the source and shines forth from us all. For every thing which is physical is a spirit, as well. The outer form changes in tune with belief and with knowledge and will, but the spirit is eternal. It springs from eternity and returns to it over and over again. It is never truly apart from it, even though we forget that and so forget how to feel that link.

Instead, we learn about the illusion of separation and time. For without time, there would be no loss as without time there would be no recovery of lost love. Without time there would be no death and no renewal. Only in time, can we experience the great pleasures and the great sorrows of love as they are expressed in this world. For life is made all the more beautiful and more tragic for the knowledge that it will someday end.

To experience extremes of joy or of terror, to feel them as one—this paradox is something which cannot be taught or learned in any conventional sense, but must be experienced to be understood. All teaching can do is point the way to the door. You must figure out how to open that door, and how to walk through to what lies on the other side. For as when the flaming doves descended upon the heads of the prophets, living representations of the fire which was stolen from the heavens long ago, you will then come to a change of perception which transforms everything and nothing at the same time. You will live in the same world as yesterday, but know it in an entirely new way, for it is you who was transformed and came to see anew.

When you experience this level of joy or of terror, when you open that door within, then you enter an altered stare of consciousness or awareness. It was once considered quite natural to be able to slip into differing and unique aspects of understanding of the world around you—especially for those of the Blood—but now most people would feel that experiencing, let alone living with, something other than the regular mundane day-to-day "natural" state of consciousness would be a bit scary, if not verging on psychotic.

We have been told quite often there is just one *right* way of seeing the world, which is why other states tend to be considered suspect, dangerous, or frivolous. This isn't true. But even though one view is not more or less real than any other, the weight of belief tends to be behind this "one consensual reality" which can make it difficult to overcome that singular viewpoint. But when we succeed in altering the way we look at the world, the world is altered as a result. How we look at the world plays a huge part in the form it takes, not just for ourselves but for those around us

Once you've achieved this altered state you can become far more aware of the connections between things, connections that generally are otherwise hidden. As a result, you may end up thinking and feeling and reacting quite differently from what some might consider normal or from what they have come to expect of you. You will also be able to do things which others might call impossible.

This is not to say that we can easily dismiss, for instance, the effects of gravity. However, if you could achieve the proper altered state of consciousness where levitation was not only possible, but even a quite normal and natural ability, and had no doubts left within you at all—a daunting prospect to be sure when you think of how much we would have to overcome to achieve that level of absolute belief—then you could, indeed, dismiss gravity and walk upon thin air. You would be existing in that moment in another state of mind, in a world where the rules are quite different than here.

There are actually stories dating back to Medieval times which speak of Saints performing miracles, including that of levitation. They would enter into an exalted state while praying and the people around them would be amazed and inspired by the sight of their feet slowly lifting off the ground until they floated free of the grip of the earth. Sadly, though, we work today not only against our own personal lack of such leaps of faith, but against the almost overwhelming weight of popular belief, a weight which tends to keep us tied firmly to the ground. The "religion" of rationalism and science has taken away our wings.

Because modern thinking does not support such beliefs or states, many other kinds of magick have to work against the weight of disbelief, too. A Witch often has to unlearn as much as he or she has learned, and then take a lot of flack for thinking outside the box, if not face accusations of being weird, odd, or downright insane. What is normal and natural for a Witch, however, is to be aware on many levels. She or he *needs* to be able to see beneath the skin of the world and be intimately aware of what forces and powers lurk in those deeper waters. A Witch has to be able to attain a state of consciousness which is not considered normal or natural by most. Though, because of the thinning of the Blood, this sort of seeing and the ability to gain and to control these sorts of altered states can be sometimes hard to achieve.

However, the world as we know it is already in the process of changing so that will change, as well. This is the time of the transformation from one Age to another, and so what has been difficult, if not nearly impossible, for the generations of the past few hundred years shall become easier in the future. It's a leap of mind, body, and spirit…but, even more so, it's a leap of the heart. For it is the heart which truly sees and the heart which really knows. Unlike the mind, a heart awakened to its true power and purpose cannot be fooled because it sees directly.

Whether we are Witches or human beings, the heart is the true center for us all. The heart is the doorway to the soul and from there the direct link back to the source from which everything springs. The mind is not the captain of the ship or the king of the castle, for the heart has that place always. Even in the Piscean Age passing away, this was a truth that was known, for there are many depictions of the "Sacred Heart of Jesus," a heart shown with a crown rising above and with thorns wrapped around it. The crown was a symbol of kingship and of the connection to the land and the people, while the thorns meant sacrifice, or making something sacred.

Your own heart is the root of who you truly are. That is the spiritual reason why heart disease is so prevalent today—for people have lost faith in themselves and deny their very essence. They do not live in their hearts, nor listen to them. If they did, then they would be more at peace with both. They would know why they are here. They would know the answer to that question which most people ask, yet rarely get answered to any satisfaction—what is the meaning of my life? And they would find their answers not in the usual place, by the "quick fix" of looking outward to buy more and more things or amass more and more money, to alcohol or drugs or food or even fixating on a job which is not their bliss and brings no real comfort, but by knowing in their heart of hearts what really matters and what really lasts. This is fulfillment and renewal of both mind and body, to find and live by joy in the spirit and trust in our essential divine natures.

There are many people today who have a spark of the old Witch Blood within them, the Blood which lived and burned in the bodies of our ancestors, the Old Ones. This spark is vibrating already to the transformations being wrought in the world as the Age changes. It shivers and shakes and resounds to each passing wave of the storm of change. This stirring, this awakening, will aid in the leap from the old world to the new, a leap which is in part a leap of perception. For as one knows and believes, so reality is changed.

The Craft is not for the weak and unwary, for greatness must always be paid for, and the token of exchange is always that which is most personal. To become an incandescent light, you must shine brightly, and where does the fuel for that come if not from the wick of your own body? But as a body burns out eventually if one is not careful, if that is the only source of fuel offered, so you must learn to feed the flame you express with the eternal spark which resides within instead. Only this will let the light shine as brightly as it can and not destroy you as a result, for the fuel will not stem from you, but from the source.

This fire, an everlasting flame which is not physical fire but the very fire of the heart, is symbolized by a crown and can be dangerous to hold onto, unless your body and mind are fit to bear it. In order to do this, you must be made pure, or when the fire of the heart comes it will burn away all remaining impurities, which can be quite a painful process to say the least. Not that it cannot be done this way, but far better to accept the flames with understanding and love already fixed firmly in your heart, than to do it with denial and fear, hoping against hope to eventually emerge whole from the other side.

To face this ordeal with pain and terror is a choice, of course, and it has been done that way many times before. To choose willingly to walk through the fire despite all your fear and let it burn away the dross of mind and flesh and emerge at the last pure of self is a great act of courage. But, equally, there is also the path of joy to pick, of braving the flames with a song on your lips and knowledge of who you are already blossoming in your heart. But this path is lesser known these days as suffering is mainly what we are taught, so much so that happiness is sometimes a harder lesson to learn and live by.

But what is purity? Unfortunately, the idea has somehow come to be mainly seen in the context of goodness in opposition to evil. Purity, however, is not meant to be what one faith or what one religion claims it to be, but is an acknowledgement rather of what is most personal and true to every single person. It is a clearing away of all that you are *not*, until all that is left is purely who you were always meant to be. It is being the bliss of your own best self, expressing the divine spark within you, letting it shine forth in the world as fully as possible.

To do this, we have to learn to really *feel* and to trust in those feelings, as we must trust in ourselves. But the problem is that most of us are afraid to feel these days. We are taught its better not to feel too much and certainly not express those feelings except to a few select friends or family, if even that. We are raised to give up dreaming as children dream, imagining as children imagine. Instead, we are taught to be rational, to be serious, to always be in control, even to pretend that we have no feelings, and so the doors close one by one, until we are prisoners behind walled fortresses, prisoners who only ever so faintly still recall the misty enchantment of the Faery realms we once knew.

We go to work and we buy things, perhaps even achieve all that society says we should desire to achieve, and yet so many of us still feel empty at times. We wander, lost in an increasingly dreary world, where each day merges into the next, with only brief glimmers of real pleasure or happiness here and there. As our news media focuses on the negative, as hatred grows, and it becomes more and more difficult to make ends meet, let alone find a life of lasting joy and accomplishment.

Part of the problem is disconnection—disconnection from ourselves, from each other, from the world. Life can easily become flat and uninteresting, and to make the world come alive again we need to learn to feel once more, to feel strongly and powerfully. But sometimes people are afraid too look too deeply, to peer behind the mask, because there may be nothing there or, worse still, a monster may be revealed. A monster of the world or, even more frightening, their own most secret monster, all that they desperately desire to keep hidden.

But the only way to face this fear is simply to face it. Because such monsters are created out of fear and despair and hatred and take their form from what is fed to them. They take the shape that we place upon them, as they live off our energies. When they are confronted and that power taken back, they can become the wellsprings they were always meant to be instead—not good, not bad, just power. As in the world at large, you have to claim and tame monsters within you in order to gain access to your own personal power.

It is then, when you exist at the center of yourself, that you are on the cusp of the past and of the future, standing in the now and yet seeing the face of eternity. Another name for this is to find your way to the mountain which is at the center of the world, around which all of time and space revolve. This spiritual mountain is the same mountain everywhere; it is the very heart of each of us, of the center of this world and all worlds, as it is the center of time and of the passing Ages.

It is on this mountain or great hill where Kings come to be crowned, the place where the earth and the sky meet and are as one. While, what lies beneath the hill is the doorway to possibility, to the Otherworld, to the realm of Faery. Where nothing is as it seems and all things are made anew. Accordingly, the treasures beneath this hill are not for the fearful of heart, nor for the small of mind. Neither gold nor silver, nor any gem of the earth, can rival what lies hidden there. At best, their sparkle is a faint echo of the glories that lie in the dark. To capture that glitter and have it for one's very own, that is why one braves the dragon. And what is the dragon if not the world monster, that which must be faced in order to gain the treasure it guards. But, in truth, that dragon is as much the treasure as that which protects the treasure, and that is why to simply slay the dragon and steal the treasure, is not enough.

This is part of the Quest. This is always part of the test. Whether you pick the path of joy or the road of terror, whether you journey by way of hardship or happiness—each having their own trials and lessons—you must face down your monster. You must brave your own dragon, in order to regain the treasure that was yours all along.

It is the same with the world treasures, for in learning how to claim our own gold, we learn how to gain the greater gold, the splendid jewels of light and the gems of powers as yet un-manifest. To go on the grand Quest for that which does not yet exist in this world, but should and must, and to face the trials given in order to bring it back, to give it a name and a form here on the Earth.

A blessed Witch is one who is in accord with their inner light and fire, who has claimed their own fate and power. They are chosen by the Gods and Goddesses to be made pure by walking the path set forth by the Divine for them to walk. They are the ones who have been made ready to journey even further, to go where few have gone in a hundred, in a thousand years, and to return home again with what is most needed, with that which will lift up the hearts of all towards the greater light. They go to seek gifts and to bring them home again.

When we dream, we wander…but what are dreams if not drifting motes of possibility? To will is to catch a piece of dream and make it real. We are the makers of this world, but a lot of us have long forgotten that, as we have forgotten ourselves. Most people say they have no such power and so deny it or, worse still, give it away to others who have no right to it or ever did. We turn away from the forces of fantasy and imagination and claim that they are just for children. But they do have power; they have the power to transform worlds, to make everything brighter and richer

The Witches were once the "Saints" of their own people. They gathered for the great feasts of old, they danced and sang and played the Game in order to work the magicks necessary to bring down the blessings of the Divine fire. They fought for the fertility of animals and of the fields, and for of all of humankind. They were the ones who were aware of the living light within them and used that light for divination and healing, to teach and to create and to walk a blessed path so that the way could be marked out for those who would come after them.

The time is now. The gates stand ready, bidding you to choose which one will be your path, to make the leap of faith into a brave new world. It's the time of awakening, both for humankind and for those Witches who have slept and forgotten for a time. It's time for those who bear the Blood to be called back to the Old Ways and to take their proper place in society once more. They are needed to fill the hollow and hurting spaces that have been left by tearing away of the Witches of old Europe, by the cutting off of Western society from its true spiritual heritage. Witches are needed to heal the wounds caused by their own lack.

Western society has been denied its own heritage and history. It has labored under an alien faith, one which does not truly speak to its ancient roots, which does not honor the beliefs which once sustained its land and people. The same beliefs which were born out of the earth and of the waters of the earth where our ancestors once walked, the birthright of field and of forest, of the fires from the heavens and of the cave of the Mothers.

Much has been lost, but nothing can ever truly be forgotten. The secrets lie within us still. They only need to be awakened once again, to be recalled, reclaimed, and renewed. For when the Blood remembers, when the doors stand open once more, when you come to stand between them as a living representative of Fire—then you are a Witch, then you are *Sorgitza*.

The Old Forest and the Old Gods

Whither shall ye walk
The straight path, the narrow path
Promising little, receiving less
The wide and roaming path
Choosing not, not to be chosen
Or the path that leads thee hither
To the kinship of the gods
That knows neither without the other
Shall ye pay their price
As they have for ye.

The Old Forest was the great wild woods which once covered a large part of Europe, though only a few small pockets of it remain today. But the Old Forest is not just a long-decimated woodland, because it is also a living memory. It is a primeval archetype within those of European descent, even if most of us do not consciously recall it much of the time. Deep down, though, we respond to the haunted and splendid majesty of such a forest when we see it in movies or in a painting or read about it in a story. It is infinitely familiar to us, despite perhaps never having visited such a forest in person.

It was into such a woods that we have known unsuspecting little girls to wander as they head off to grandmother's house, only to find a big bad wolf barring their path. It was under the shade of those great trees that knights of old ventured in search of dragons, fair maidens, and endless adventure. For the greenwoods have long called to both the brave and the foolhardy, the hungry and the hopeless, whether drawn into its verdant shadows by dancing lights, tales of ancient treasures, or by the ever so brief glimpse of some gleaming smoke-pale stag.

This is the forest of fable and fairytale, of story and dream, enchanted and haunted and home to great danger and great beauty alike. It is a holy place, filled with sacred springs and secret caves, where groves of ancient oaks rise up to form the first "cathedrals," some of them so large that they came to be known as King Oaks, father-oaks whose roots are fed by the very wellsprings of power in the land. For the Old Forest had a life and spirit all its' own, one that our ancestors were intimately aware of and sought to live in accord with.

It's because of this deep and sacred memory that so many fantasy stories and fairytales take place in some sort of magickal forest. This forest comes from the knowledge that we all share, from the silent remembering that is ingrained within our bodies, within our very blood and bone. Why this is so is not just because our ancestors once lived in or near the Old Forest, but because such a forest—primitive, powerful, home to mystery and terror alike—is part of who we are, of where we come from. Such forests existed long before there was any written language.

So, it isn't just the Old Forest of a long-ago Europe that we recall in our dreams and stories. It is the forests that we all knew ages ago, long before the rise of civilization, from a time when we were much more in tune with the land and saw ourselves as a part of it, the same as the trees and the rocks and the animals. That sort of animistic, magickal thinking was how our ancestors saw the world—a world animated by spirits of all kinds— and which has come down to us as the idea of a haunted forest, one full of specters and ghosts and elves and faeries.

But even if we only remember the Old Forest, the forest primeval, in our dreams and fairytales, the forest certainly remembers us. The trees remember who we are and what we once were, for they pass down the knowledge from one growth to another. They are, themselves, yet in touch with and a part of the first forest that ever rose upon the ashes created by the birth of the Earth. The only ones who can recall even older things are the rocks and stones, the very bones of the Earth Mother.

To all such spirits of the Earth, we are but a passing glimmer, a flash of light, a sudden and electrifying spark, for we are as quick as they are long. Our time upon this planet has been brief by their reckoning, so we are considered by them to be very like children, children who have a lot to learn yet. This can make Earth spirits, of all the spirits we interact with, some of the hardest for us to relate to and understand. Though, understand them we must, as best we can, in order to understand our own past and where we all came from.

All expression has its reflection and its echo, so that when something exists—most especially a supremely powerful something—it casts ripples of itself out in every direction, including the past and of the future. The Old Forest, then, is in some fashion the same primeval first forest, as it is also a shade of the great forests which shall rise again in the far flung future. They are linked together by the initial creation, the initial thought, and by the idea of each other, thus reflecting the circular nature of the universe.

For all that falls, rises again—Witches, the great forest of legend, the Old Gods—as magicks and mysteries lie fallow and hidden for a time, for a winter of the soul, only to sprout and vine and blossom and bloom once more into springtime. The past is the seed for the future, as the future is the spark for the past. So the Old Forest has been lost, but yet it has never been lost, for it lingers inside each and every one of us who can claim descent from its wild lands. And it is there, within that forest, within the stories of that forest, that we can find our beginnings again. As we can find our old Gods.

But just who are these old Gods? Where have They been? And why are They now returning to us?

The Gods of the *Sorgitza*, of the Old Forest, form an archaic Witch pantheon. However, They are also Gods Who have had many names in countless lands and over many generations. The names that They have given to be used in this book are but of the few that They have known over the years. For example, the Goddess of the West, Ariadne, has also been known of old as Aphrodite and Cerridwen, as well as the Lady of the Lake.

The same is true for the Gods who appear in this book; some of Their names will sound familiar, such as Tehot—which is a name that comes out of ancient Egypt, though He Himself is far older even than that—and some will not. An additional example would be Ahkenahmnos, the God of the South-West, who once was also known as Dionysus, the God of the wild-haired Maenads, His Priestesses of old.

But even if a particular name They choose to use now is unfamiliar to us—being a name so old that it has all but been forgotten or, conversely, a very new one—Their inner natures yet remain true to who They are. The essence of who They are does not change, though minor aspects of Their character and Their names may alter over time and from one land to the next. As one attribute of Their nature may be the primary focus for a particular era or a particular country, then become secondary for another.

For example, the South Goddess, the Goddess of Fire, once had as Her symbol a stone spire and now—for the Aquarian Age—Her symbol has become a circle of raised candles. On the surface, it may seem that a spire and a circle of lifted candles has very little to do with each other, but when put together with an understanding of what She is like, what Her nature is, there is a symbolism shared between them. For as a spire of stone reaches towards the sky and brings down the power of the heavens, so too does a circle of raised candles accomplish much the same purpose, even though no longer fashioned of stone, but of living flesh and flame. So the great cathedrals of the future shall not be made of brick or of metal or stone, but of the very people themselves.

The question may be asked, though, as to just why the Gods of the Old Forest should find Themselves here in the Americas as well as in Europe? It is for the simple reason that They journeyed here with us, with the descendants of those who once knew and worshipped Them. As we traveled across the ocean to the New World, our beliefs, our stories and memories, whether conscious or not, came with us. Our very blood brought with us the ways and secrets of the Old Ones, as they were in our hearts, in our spirits, just as the spirit of the Old Forest lingers there, ready to take root again.

Of course, the lands here in this country have their own stories, their own spirits, their own Gods. So it is important that, as we learn to live in accord with the Earth here, that the Gods of the Old World commune in peace with the spirits who already reside here in the New. It is vital that their old Gods and our old Gods come to an accord and be united in common purpose, which is the fertility and vitality of this land and all who live here. As we may also forge our own link to the land and spirits here, if we open our hearts and make them welcome. If we honor and respect them and mingle together our blood and bone, as was done in the past, making us one with the Earth.

When we and the Old Gods are linked to the Earth—to its sacred places, its wellsprings of power—our fates are then woven together...land, Gods, Witches, and people. So it was in the old days and so it will be again. For Their prosperity is our prosperity, as ours is Theirs. Even if we have wandered far, we can return home yet again. We can rebuild our foundation, reawaken to our world, to our powers, to ourselves. We can take the teachings of the past and soar into the future upon the wings which the Old Ones once knew and which we now know is as much our heritage as the Blood.

The great and haunted forests of our hearts' desire, the rising crown of stars, each flame a soul...what is the Craft? What is the Blood? It is a web, a tapestry, a wheel, a song, a dream, a Quest, the Phoenix spiraling upwards from the ashes of its own fiery destruction again and again, just as Witches rise and spin and spark and spiral, Shining Ones all.

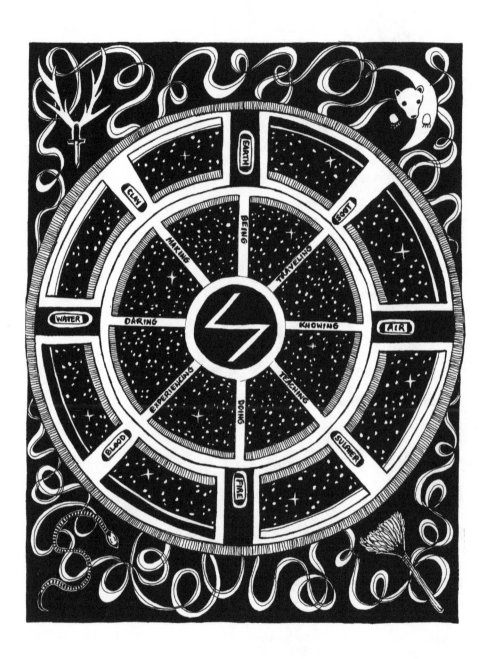

80

Part Two

The Gods of the Old Forest

*What is woven is always woven in three, for this was the form Fate chose of old to show Her works in—the weavers who sit within the dark, blind to all, yet all-seeing, and they are three, always three, yet ever and always one. This was stolen by the worshippers of the God of dust and storms, of the cup and the cross, for they would have their God **be** Fate, but Fate is no main nor ever was, just as it is no woman, nor ever could be.*

Fate is only a seeming of three wrinkled faces in the dark, one to spin and one to weave and one to cut. Though there is yet another old face for those who have eyes to see her, the face of all the empty spaces, that which is also spun and woven and cut into the fabric of all that is. The shadow that is not a shadow for it is and is not at the same time.

She is riddle and what lies between time and space, and the hidden echo in the words of prayer cast to the sky. I speak of Her for I am near to Her, yet not of Her, for I have a face and a name and so am not shadow. But if you wish to speak to Her, speak to me and She shall hear. Just as She shall hear if you speak to the Earth, to the oldest ones of all.

Some things are not meant to be named—mark this well, for your kind is much in love with the dream that all may be known, all may be named. Children of Adam, you imagine his gift your own, but as Adam was not a man so men bear not his gift, and even Adam dared not name the nameless ones, the great hollows and echoing expanses of all that cannot enter into the smallness of this world without sundering it forever.

Dream small dreams. The larger shall come in time, when you have learned the lessons of the light, the teachings of the dark, and whither to walk upon the turbulent

81

web, the distant most stars. I am Destiny. I say you shall walk there in time, though that time is not yet now. Your choice, but the wiser one would be to heed my warnings and my blessings, for I have set this web upon your heart as well as on the heavens, so that each shall reflect the other.

Circe, the Goddess of Destiny

The Quarters

To North and South
To East and West
We've wandered
To the one we love the best—
The lord of our hearts
His heat desire
The lady of our flesh
Who courts with fire.

North, East, South, and West are the four Quarters and each of these Quarters has their attendant God and Goddess, one of which represents the physical element and one the spiritual or metaphysical element. In the case of the Quarters, the Goddess is the physical element of Earth, of Air, of Fire, or of Water, while the God represents the aspects of Being, Knowing, Doing, and Daring. When combined They make up the totality of the Quarter.

This is the first crossroads, a crossroads that is made up of the Four which is also Eight, and formed the very foundation of being. It does not matter where you live or in what direction water may lie or deserts or mountains, for these elements and the paths along which they pass came long before the geography we know today. They are pathways that lie within us, for we also stand at the center of the Four and have our beginnings in them.

North is Earth and Being.
East is Air and Knowing.
South is Fire and Doing.
West is Water and Daring.

The North is also linked to Midsummer, to the high places and the height of summer and of the earthly King's power. While, the South is Midwinter, the cave from which the light is born again to the world, the silence that awaits midnight on the longest night in the year. Accordingly, East is the dawn and Spring Equinox, the rising of the morning star and the blossoming of new life. As West is dusk, twilight, and the Autumnal Equinox, the sacrifice and the harvest as one, sowing the seeds for the next cycle to begin again.

The North

Slow time
Stone time
We walk upon the bones of the past
The bones of the dead
Their mouths are open
Their hands closed
Upon the roots of the earth
Blue seed necklaces and bands
Of mottled white snakeskin
As flowers died to mark their passage
From one birth to the next
When will it begin?

North is Earth and the caves of the Earth, the secret birthing place. It is the darkness from which all come, from where all are born to the world of light. The beings of the North are those who keep vigil, who watch over us all.

The Watchtower of the North is a tall, thin spire that stands over a vast field of ice, stone, and stillness. It stands in the middle of a cold land, blue and silver-grey as if made of long frozen tears. The Tower there is less a tower than a mountain rising up in a thin sharp spike as if formed of liquid stone caught in the quiet of the eternal. A tower made of the risen bones of the living rock, a tower formed of vibrant crystal that holds sounds that no one living can hear.

Inside the tower, a round room holds a white mushroom-shaped table, but as to what rests upon the table…few can see and even fewer understand, for it is not a thing of mind or of eye, but pure Being. A plate, a shield, a chessboard, a web—what lies on the table is many things and yet none at all.

The Tower of the North is all this and more.

North is that which turns so very fast, that it no longer moves at all. North is the place of mystery and of beginnings, hence it is where those who seek the Gods, those who seek themselves, must go in the end to learn the very riddle of Being. To wake and to never sleep, each moment of time immobile, yet ever changing. There voices rise up to make no sound.

The Gate of the Gods can only be opened if you know all of what you are, all of the names that you have claimed, and all of the forms that you have worn. The quiet Earth is as much a grave as a place of birth, but unless you know the silence within you cannot hold tight to both at the same time and come into the wisdom of Being.

Earth

Ardwena is the Goddess of the North, the Goddess of the Earth. She is a Goddess in whose honor the bones and skull of bears were once placed in the deepest caves to be worshipped. Her home was the Old Forest which remains today only in secluded pockets, one of which is the Ardennes. Ardwena is in Her own words the *"Goddess of children, of the Ardennes, and of the Danube river,"* the Danube being a traditional wellspring of power.

She is a Goddess of motherhood, of children, one who fiercely protects Her family. She is an Old One Herself, a Goddess who recalls when the world was young. She knew the oldest of all Witches, back before Rome was even a city, when Egypt was still at its height and power. She knows the old ways of working magick, the old rites lost even by the Witches themselves. Rites that She is willing to teach if you can convince Her that you are open to being taught and willing enough to learn. In this, Her patience is long, but not eternal, and She does not suffer fools, though She may be charmed by an honest heart and a kind smile.

She prefers to do things Her way, which are the old ways, and often feels that today's Witches and today's methods are too much driven by our heads and not by our hearts. She feels that we are not in accord with the needs and rhythms of our own bodies, and so much of what we do makes no sense anymore.

Ardwena is the Goddess whose essence can be seen in the old rounded stone statues discovered by archaeologists, emblems of female fertility. She is always and ever of the Earth and the spirits of the Earth are Hers to know and care for. She knows of old things, of the old ways when humankind was young. So if you wish to learn of how things were done thousands of years ago, of what Witches once were and what they could do then—you should call upon Ardwena to teach you:

Lahmahk Ardwena
Lahmahk Ardwena Itzah
Arhdwena
Ensieta
Arahnak
Arahnak

In order to know Her best, She tells us that *"there is power in the land, in the old places. To know Ardwena, you must touch the land. You must go into the land. The earth spirits are different from land to land, but all earth spirits flow into Ardwena… earth spirits go from the land, they go into the land and return. When Witches put blood into the land, it wakes the earth spirits. When Witches die, they are buried and the earth spirits return…to wake the earth spirits is to know Ardwena…to call Ardwena is through the land…arahnak, arahnak, arahnak…nlame ru vashle…do not forget, do not forget, tell sleeping Witches do not forget. Too much is forgotten. Do not forget."*

To aid in awakening the land, Ardwena tells us that female Witches should bury their moon blood within the land that they wish to be a part of. This both serves to awaken the Earth spirits and to form a bond with that particular piece of land, so that Witches will be drawn back to it both in their travels and when they are reborn once more to this world from the other. While to best come to know Ardwena Herself, Witches need to Dance the Blood as much as possible.

Her Sabbats are Midsummer and Lammas. Her symbol is the earth, a stone, a bear, or a stone carved or painted with a bear.

Invocation of Ardwena

You may use a stone or a stone carved into the likeness of a bear or painted with the symbol of a bear. Have the Priestess being invoked into stand to the North of the circle if possible, with her arms crossed over her chest. The Priest invokes with a wand carved or painted like a snake, or by raising the bear or stone up in front of her, saying:

Old one
Ancient of days
She of the caves
Of the great bear of the sky
Thee we invoke
Thee we charge to appear before us
By earth and by stone
Thee we invoke
Ardwena, Ardwena, Ardwena
Enter into
The body of your Priestess (name)
Who awaits thee.

The Priestess should open her arms for the Priest to touch the bear or stone to her stomach, over her womb. If She desires to take the bear or stone, give it to Her to hold.

Alternate Invocation of Ardwena

By the cave of the Mothers
By the bones and skull
Of the great bears of old
Thee we call
By the wellspring
The wild river
And the stone altar
In the depths of the mountains
In the heart of the great forest
Thee we invoke
Lady of earth
And of the spirits of the earth
Ardwena Ardwena Ardwena

Enter into
The body of your Priestess (name)
Who awaits thee.

Being

The God of the North is Eahnos. He is generous and kindly and forgiving and one of His symbols is the cornucopia for He gives all in abundance. Eahnos stands at the North, but He looks in two directions at the same time. He looks to the East and He looks to the West, to the past and to the future, to both time and eternity. He is the gateway through which the stillness of the North flows and has long been a God of doors and of hinges. Unsurprisingly then, one of His other names is Janus. He is also the God of hills, pyramids, mountains, and ziggurats.

Eahnos is the God of silence. A whisper begins. A whisper ends. It is the same whisper from start to finish, while the silence that falls between is the shadow of the sound. So it is with Eahnos, for though He looks to the past and to the future, He also sees in every way it is possible to see. He knows male and female, night and day, up and down, all that springs from the eternal now into the world of time and mankind; He sees that though they are two, they are one at the same time.

He is not just a God who stands in the doorway, but is the doorway Himself. Through Eahnos pours forth all that is possible. But as it is difficult for great powers to pass whole and entire into the land of form and time, so some may only make a foothold here. Some may but peer at us through a living mask, for to behold them in their true and complete aspect would result in pain, madness, and even death. For such was the fate of Zeus's lover when she asked Him to show Himself to her in His full might and glory and He, having sworn to grant her what she most desired, could not dissuade her. So He appeared to her and she was burnt to ashes and He could but rescue their immortal child from what little remained.

So, the great powers, the great Gods, dare not show Their true face to us while we exist here in the fragile flesh, for to do so is to risk much. But yet we may catch glimpses of those powers in the shapes and masks that they adorn Themselves with when They enter into our world. Though, to do so, They must pass through the North Gate and take on the limitations of age and fate.

In this way is Eahnos is a "father" to us all. He is father to all that pours into the world from the unseen realms. He is the spiritual source and archetype of what has come down to us as "Father Time, " "Father Christmas," and, of course, "Santa Claus." Small wonder then, that Old St Nick or Santa is said to live at the North Pole. While, the image of the wise old wizard is also based upon him, as well as the jolly giver of all good things, the Lord of the Horn of Plenty. In this, He is less the God upon the mountaintop as He is the mountain itself, that which connects the roots of the earth to the sky. The hill that holds within it the hidden treasures, that have yet to find their way into the world above.

The spirits of Being and of silence are of Him, the silence that echoes the song. The silence, from which the song is born, the song which made all things for the dawn. In that way, they are not so much silent beings, but are of a song so great that its entirety cannot be heard, a song that has gone so far beyond that it has turned into the essence of silence itself. This is the same riddle as that of movement of the North—when what moves turns so very fast that it no longer moves at all.

The spirits of Being are the least knowable, for they are close to the source, to the still point where the universal spirit pours into the world we all live in. They exist in the in-drawn breath, the quiet moment where neither thought nor motion is considered. It is hard for us beings of time to be silent and still, and so it is hard for us to connect to them. We are far too young to have learned the pure being that is required—to move so fast and sing so purely that no movement and no sound remains.

Eahnos asks us *"what is it you require when all is given? Look around you, look inside you, and you will see. Bounty immeasurable. All that is required and more. Children you are and as children you need to see, you must believe. For who are we but those who have given you life and love you best of all."*

His Sabbats are Midwinter, the silent midnight of the longest darkness of the year, and Lammas. His symbols are a pyramid, a ziggurat, and a bull's horn.

Invocation of Eahnos

Priest stands to the North with his hands crossed over his chest. Priestess invokes with snake wand or a bull's horn, saying:

Bahgahbe Lahkah Bahkahbay
Lahmahk Kahi Ardutin
Lahmahk Sahmahk Famyolas
Sahmahk Kahi Ertahlia
Ertahlia

Eahnos can only be properly invoked in these words. You may also choose to hand Him the bull's horn at this point, or perhaps a representation of a cornucopia.

The East

Light as thistledown
Witches whirl in the wind
How can they fly so high?
They are light of heart and mind
And their souls are made of air
And moonlight
That's how
They believe
And are one with the sky.

East is Air and Knowing, free and full of the hope of the dawn. The air is bright dreams and infectious laughter, playfulness and teasing delight. Breath is air is mind is flesh of the spirits. Air is knowing what is to be known and so it can be said that "a little birdie told me so," for birds ride the winds and go where they go and partake of their nature. Birds are messengers between the earth and the skies, between man and the Divine. Doves, eagles, ravens, kites, kestrels, geese, robins, wrens—they all travel between worlds and carry back messages.

One of the first kings of old was a hawk, a crowned prince upon the rich banks of the Nile, so all would know his place in the order of things. Just as it is no coincidence that a bird's quill was once used in writing. Nor, that angels take feathered flight upon the clouds, that holy men were painted as walking upon the air, or faeries are portrayed as being adorned with the gossamer wings of splendid butterflies. These are all emblems of the Eastern horizon, of both Air and Knowing.

The Gate of Faery lies to the East, the doorway to the realm of the winds. This is the realm where that which is can shift in accord with a change in the air, where roads lead in many directions. The magicks here are not

Witch magicks, for they rely less on will and concentration than on wit and laughter. What matters most to walk this Gate is a certain lightness of the soul, so that the body may fly as upon a dust mote. Here, you must be light as thistledown, light enough for a puff of air to carry you up amongst the clouds, where you can the Earth beneath you as though it were a compass map.

The Watchtower of the East is spiral, a glass horn of wonder and enchantment to pierce the dome of the skies, a tower floating between heaven and earth almost as if in a dream. Pearl and bone and shining clear, it is strong and solid one moment and misty as a ghost the next. It is both there and not there, material and ethereal, real and a riddle. This is the same glass that was once also gold, the gold of a poor lost slipper. As Cinderella was a phoenix, a child of the dawn and of the ash, half as much a Faery as her own godmother.

The Tower of Air is a spiraling ivory unicorn's horn. It is made of wish and dream and the desire to touch what lies just beyond the mirror. It's the same tower that appears in the far mists fairytales, one that recedes the closer you draw near to it. Birds fly about this tower, birds that are not birds, and the air is filled with whispers and sounds that no mortal mouth, nor throat can make.

Every little girl dreams at least once of the gleaming castle of the Faery princess, and their dreams mold the Tower of the East much as their dreams are touched by those smooth glimmering walls and by a sprinkle of fallen pixie dust. Which is not to imply that the East and that the Eastern Tower is nothing but sweetness and light, fun and fancy, for the East can be stern and it can be sharp, as laughter may sting even more deeply than the most finely honed blade.

The Eastern Tower is all this and more.

The East is of the floating spirits of the Air, those who have been called elves or Faery or Fey. As they have been named the Gentry, the Fair Ones, the Sidhe, and the Seelie Court, from which we get our modern word "silly," though it is not a silliness that comes through a lack of understanding of the workings of the world, but by truly seeing them in their greater light. However, none of these names are their true names, for we cannot speak their language and so cannot pronounce what they call themselves.

The Lady of Air and dawn lives within Her spirits; they are a part of Her and She is a part of them, as they are all part of the winds. Hers are the white flowers of May, the petals of joy. As Her consort wears the black flowers of October, the blossoms of fear and those who come at midnight, in a rush, in a horde.

Her name is Arien and She is a springtime Goddess, a Goddess of laughter and riddles and games. Both Her blood and the blood of Her children is white, pure joy, and their eyes are pure black, the black of the empty spaces between the stars. It was their blood which fell from the sky and painted the red mushroom in the forests of the most ancient Earth, creating the food that sets the spirit free to walk the realms of night.

A white cake spotted with blood is one mystery and a red cake spotted with white is another, but they are mirrors of each other as Her spirits are mirrors of Witches. Here you find one hand reaching out to another across worlds, where crossed arms, crossed wrists, and the meeting of eyes become a promise and a pledge, the same promise and pledge that joined Witches and the Faery folk thousands of years ago.

Arien is the Goddess of East and of the Air and She is eager to see new faces and to receive and answer questions. She is the Faery Queen of old, both beautiful and tricksy in nature. She says to us *"ask, ask, ask—you don't have questions? You don't seek to know the very secrets of the universe? Others are less shy and they come to us and plead…tell us, show us, let the winds come and blow through our souls, leaving behind such messages as have been rarely seen or heard before. But we, we are family and who better to share secrets with, to keep them with, to laugh and sing and fEast with? We, we are family even when it is you who forget and cover your eyes, press your hands to your ears and sing nah, nah…it is only we, we are here alone, all alone. But I say and you shall hear all the same, no, it is not true. It is not true and never has been."*

Her Sabbats are Spring Equinox and Beltane and Her symbol is the besom, or broom, though a feather will do, as well.

Invocation of Arien

Priestess being invoked into stands in the East if possible, with hands crossed over her chest. A broom is raised before her, handle end down, as Priest invokes:

Laughing one
Sister to the stars
And to the whirling madness
By the breath of incense
Thee we invoke
Thee we charge to appear before us
By the sweet rush of the winds
Thee we invoke
Arien, Arien, Arien
Enter into
The body of your Priestess (name)
Who awaits thee.

Broom is then held to body of Priestess and the Goddess may take it for Her own.

Alternative Invocation of Arien

Bright lady
Blessed one of the dawn
Queen of the air
By joy and love and laughter
Thee we invoke
By the whir and rush and whirl
Of the winds
We call thee
Oh shining one
By the riddle of the stars
And by storm and delight
Thee we call
Arien Arien Arien
Enter into
The body of your Priestess (name)
Who awaits thee.

Knowledge comes in its own time. If you try to seize knowledge before you are ready to receive it, it will not be knowledge, but illusion. It will be like Faery gold that turns to dust when you return to the land above or pixie dust in a bottle that cannot make anyone fly, no matter how hard they try. For knowledge stolen without care or concern, can turn and burn the hand of those who grasp it and conjure from the darkness the very demons and shadowkin that lurk within us all.

Many say the East is "thought," but that is not strictly so. The East is Knowing. The kind of Knowing that comes upon one in a sudden rush, sure and powerful and true, and that owes its strength not to any human thought nor page within a book nor any argument ever made. It's not the sort of understanding born of book learning or the long drawn-out processes of logical thought—but an inherent and immediate understanding that stems from the soul. It's the "Eureka!" moment.

Seeking knowledge, teaching and learning do not belong to the East, for they are actions and so are part of the South and the South-East. The Knowing of the East does not *do*, it simply *is*. This is true knowledge. Knowledge that is neither learned nor earned, but is like a window suddenly opening up in your mind, in your heart, revealing connections and insights that normally go unseen and unacknowledged.

The spirits of Knowing are not human and do not perceive the world or the workings of the world as humans do. They may even seem indifferent at times, but that is because what they see as "good"—and by good they mean what is right and correct—may be incomprehensible to us who have a more short term or limited view. These spirits are not bad or needlessly cruel, but they are "alien" to us in a lot of ways.

Tehot is the God of the East and of Knowing and He knows all. He is ready to hear any questions you may seek to pose him, though you must be careful how and what it is that you ask. Sometimes, His answers may sound like riddles, but they are not. It is simply that the question you pose may not be answered truthfully except in a way that does not fit into normal human language or linear understanding. Most modern languages are not constructed in a manner which easily handles expression of the greater truths. Not surprisingly, then, some of His answers but inspire more questions.

Tehot was a God known to ancient Egypt, but He is far older than that. When first a word, a name, was spoken and so called that thing into being... Tehot was there. He is the lord of language, of that ultimate connection between the name and what is named. And so magicians of the past used His aid in the creation of their spells.

Tehot should be invoked when the Priest is seated, preferably cross-legged, for this is the pose of the ancient scribe. He will not mind if you write or take notes while conversing with Him, for writing is something He is understandably fond of. He also enjoys being asked questions, but it is a good idea to figure out ahead of time the exact phrasing of what you wish to ask Him.

His Sabbats are Autumn Equinox and Beltane and He is best invoked with sweet incense, though you may also choose to use paper or parchment and a writing utensil, such as a quill. Though, since Tehot is well aware of the passage of time, you can also use a pen of some sort.

Invocation of Tehot

Priest being invoked into seats himself on floor or ground to the East of the circle, cross-legged if possible. A censor of smoking incense may be used to invoke His presence, with a quill or other writing utensil if desired. The Priest may rest his arms upon his crossed legs as invocation is read:

Chariot of knowledge
Brother of tomorrow
By the name and by the word
Of riddle and creation
Thee we invoke
Thee we charge to appear before us
By sweet smelling incense
Thee we invoke
Tehot, Tehot, Tehot
Enter into
The body of your Priest (name)
Who awaits thee.

The Priestess raises the censor of incense and gently blows the smoke into the Priest's face. She may also hand Him the quill or pen at this time.

Alternate Invocation of Tehot

Oh song of glory
Oh pledge and word of light
By the sands of history
By the seeing glass of time
I invoke thee
By all that is veiled
And by all that may be revealed
I invoke thee
Tehot
Lord of knowledge
Of the patterns writ upon the sky
And upon the trembling earth
Oh brother of the dawn
I call thee
Tehot Tehot Tehot
Speak now through your Priest (name)
Answer what we would ask
Of thee.

The South

One hand clasps another.
We spiral and spin, a dance that recalls the forces of life and creation.
It is no mistake, no coincidence, no haphazard meeting place we attend…for we have
come to make the center and to re-make what was un-made, to set it in place and start
it all whirling again.

One hand clasps another.
The power passes between us, growing as it spins, as it spirals.
We are as much a part of it as it is of us.

To believe in the fire is to let it reside in your hearts, to be a part of the first force of
life, that which raged across the sky and tumbled out the stars.

The South is the place of Fire and of Doing.

The South is also the proper quarter of all Witches because when the Blood
is stirred to wakefulness and awareness it is a bright flame, a shining star.
Witches are meant to be Shining Ones and the patterns that they weave are
in remembrance of the patterns woven by the stars in the heavens. For the
fire in the Blood is the same fire as that of the distant stars, just as Witches
are seeds from the stars, seeds that have been sown in the fertile Earth.

Far, far to the South is the Watchtower of the South, wherein the illuminated
ones wait for those who find their way to their realm. They are beings of
Fire, for they have fully awoken to the secret of their true nature; that they
and the stars are one. Theirs is the diadem of jewels, each gemstone that
of crystallized light. Theirs also is the long hallway lined with mirrors,
each mirror a door, and the cup that holds the seed of infinite possibility.

The South Tower contains the forge, as well, though what the forge creates it cannot long contain. Weapons of light and of fire are made here, as well as moon crowns and rings of gold. It is here that the company gathers, those whose hearts and will have passed through the center of the forge's flames and been made anew. They who have been tempered and honed, until they shine with a glory all their own.

This Tower is of a black stone that is also black metal, the sort that once fell from the skies. Sometimes, it still glows with the red heat of that descent, recalling its own origin. The room in the center of the tower contains the cup, the famed cup of legend and of delight. This cup is made of both gold and silver intermingled, and yet of a metal as yet unknown to man. Though the cup appears different for everyone, just as each blade forged is unlike the next and the last.

Gems and pearls and golden treasure beyond measure lie here, with a dragon curled about the root of the tower to keep guard. To walk through the door of the tower is to walk through the dragon's mouth, and few prove themselves brave enough at the last to dare its fangs, let alone its fiery breath. Every scale upon the dragon is a reflection of a soul of those who have passed through and those yet to come.

The Tower of the South is all this and more.

The beings of the Fire may be called the *illuminare*, though they have had other names, and are, according to the Goddess of the East, those who "*ate the fire.*" The *illuminare* may also be called the "ascended masters." They are beings of Fire; they burn with a pure white light for this same light has consumed them. This is a consummation that they sought out because they desired to be burnt, leaving only the pure spark that lies are the core of all things and all beings.

The *illuminare* are not those who are illuminated, but those who illuminate. They wait for us to come to them, for they shall not come to us first. It is part of the test. Can you go outward enough—or inward enough—in order to find them, in order to find yourself? Can you pass the tests required along the way, for there are always tests, there is always an ordeal. The masters are those who have mastered their own selves and so know the truth about themselves. They *live* in their own Self, in their own hallway of mirrors and doors, wherein lies the cup that grants eternal life. A cup filled with a single pearl that is the first metaphor, the seed of truth, and from which all pours forth.

Fire

The Goddess of Fire is Sahlonshai. She is also the Goddess of the Priesthood, of Priests and Priestesses throughout time. For this Age, She is the Priestess of Ahtahmenak, who is the Light Bearer. According to Her own words, She carries *"the light and life before Him, so that all may see that these are His gifts. I bear the torch lit from the fire stolen from the Gods, given to Man that they may be as one with the Gods…"*

She is the Seeing, Speaking, and Oneness: *sahl-on-shai*. She is the peace within the heart of the raging fire, within the center of the whirling tide, and She was known in the past as Salame, Salaam, and Shalom. She is the eye of the storm and the heart of the Phoenix. As the Light Bearer is the burning fire of enlightenment, so She is the calm core at the very center of that burning.

Hers is the dance which reveals, the spinning whirlwind of flame around the quiet center which is Her own gift. For She is the quietude, the stillness in the middle of madness, though the precise nature of Her peace changes. For Sahlonshai changes as the Ages change, as the world's Priests and Priestesses must change to best minister to that Age. As the flame of each year, of each Age, leaps into the next, so the form that expresses that flame also alters and shifts. A new Phoenix rises, a new Priesthood rises, new patterns emerge, and so the Goddess of the South, of the Fire of life and of the Blood, is born to a new name.

She is the lady of the tower, of the torch, of temple and sanctuary, of each and every holy place. She is the Queen of prayers, of the round of roses, of beaded meditation, and the breath which whispers promises and pleas to the Gods. Whenever a candle is lit in the name of the Divine, She is there. Hers is the way of ritual. Hers is the calling and the vocation—that which speaks directly to the heart and summons those who are needed to take up the mantle of the Priesthood. Of primary importance, She says to be a true Priest or a Priestess you *"must do."*

She also tells us that Hers is *"the kiss that falls to the cup, the blood that falls from the cup, the life that comes from the blood, the kiss that comes with the life."*

104

Her Sabbats are Midwinter and Imbolc and Her symbol is a raised candle or a circle of raised candles.

Invocation of Sahlonshai

The Priestess should stand to the South of the circle if possible with her hands crossed over her chest. Priest or all in circle may lift lit candles on high to invoke. Priest may also use snake wand to invoke while all others in circle hold up lit candles.

Priestess of the ages
Maiden Mother
Tender lady of the tower
And of the brightest temple
Thee we invoke
Thee we charge to appear before us
Oh blessed one
Thee we invoke
Sahlonshai, Sahlonshai, Sahlonshai
Enter into
The body of your Priestess (name)
Who awaits thee.

Priest offers a lit candle to the Priestess.

Alternative Invocation of Sahlonshai

Lady of peace
Keeper of the shroud
And of the cup
The prayer of the flame
Within the flesh
Within the bone
Thee we invoke
Sahlonshai
By the dancers in the temple
Whose feet weave patterns
Of life and death and light
By the pledge that reaches to the heaven

By the song of delight
Thee we invoke
Oh blessed one of the God
Thee we call
Sahlonshai Sahlonshai Sahlonshai

Doing

The God of the South is Tzahranos. He is a God of fertility and of life's renewal, and can be seen in the summer storm, particularly in the bolt of lightning that lances down to connect the earth and the sky. His symbol is the snake, for the snake sheds its skin and is reborn again and again.

Tzahranos is the whipcord, the strike of the serpent, the tongue of the heavens. His power lies between the oak and the sky, in the arch and spit and spark of the lightning bolt which ties them together. His is the raised pole of the May around which tender maidens come to dance, to weave their patterns through the power of desire. His is the tree of sacrifice and renewal, the center pole that is both the rainbow and the snake.

He is the lord of the fields, of the orchards and of the Blood. It is He who raises His open hands to the sky when He comes to the mountains, to the tallest peak in the land. He lifts His face to the sun, the sun which is also His symbol and which forms His crown, a crown made of berries red as blood and of the golden leaves of life's victory. He is Kingship and the understanding of Kingship which is love, the kind of love that fulfills and sacrifices of itself to give for renewal ever and again. In this, He is the anointed one and best beloved of the Earth and of the Earth Goddess, Ardwena.

Tzahranos is also the God of Doing, which is the inherent nature of all Witches. His is the world of action, for if one is to be a proper Priest or Priestess then one *must* act. For words count for little when they are not matched by deeds, as magick is not enough without the preparation in the physical world for the results of that magick, the same way that a seed must be sown in rich ground for it to take root and prosper.

He says to us *"laugh to know me, live to find me. I am in you as you are in me. I am all you are, all you were, all you will be so long as there is breath in your bodies and fire in your hearts. I am unquenchable. I am the taste found in every raised cup and upon every shared plate, for I am upon the vine and upon the stalk, in every field and forest and upon every branch. Dance, sing, make merry of all of life's pleasures, for this is the fEasting that I grant, that I have made my sacrifice for. A willing enough sacrifice it must be said, for mine is the way of sacrifice and the way of joy in sacrifice, the way of generation and of regeneration, of home and heart and hearth and harvest. I am the seed. I am the green. I am the golden wheat of heaven. I am the crown of life's promise."*

His Sabbats are Midsummer and Imbolc. His symbol is the snake or wand, or a wand carved or painted as a snake. A lightning bolt or a stalk of wheat can also be used.

Invocation of Tzahranos

Priest stands to the South of the circle if possible, hands crossed over his chest. Priestess invokes with raised snake or lightning wand or some stalks of wheat or other grain, saying:

By the golden crown of the sun
The living light
The seed within
And the seed without
Thee we invoke
Thee we charge to appear before us
Oh lord of life
Thee we invoke
Tzahranos, Tzahranos, Tzahranos
Enter into
The body of your Priest (name)
Who awaits thee.

Priestess should lay the snake wand vertically on Priest's chest, the head of the snake uppermost, or hand him the wheat or grain.

Lord of the fields
Of flocks and herds and love
By what is planted
And what is sown
By the blessings of the sun
Thee we invoke
Tzahranos
Great one of the fertile cross
Of the sacred oak of kings
The fall and rise
The seed of sacrifice
The renewal of days
The rush of desire
We call thee
Tzahranos Tzahranos Tzahranos
Enter into
The body of your Priest (name)
Who awaits thee.

The West

Green-eyed willow why
Bend thee to the well side
Red and yellow ribbons tied
For the luck that's there
Grey-fingered willow knows
Seek the way the waters go
Cast a charm and will it so
But only if you dare

The West is Water and Daring. It is the source of creation and destruction, the restless ocean from which ideas spring, as water flows and moves and transforms what it touches. Together with Earth, it makes up the physical components of us all; it forms the clay that will be imparted with breath and the spark of life.

The West represents unknown vistas and mysteries as yet unexplored, that which can be brought to form and realization by those who dare to go down into the depths. Some of what is brought forth from the deeps are actual physical, material things, while others remain ideas, though ideas can, of course, change the world. In this way, Water is not just feeling and Daring, but is inspiration and the place where legends are first conceived of.

Water is a major part of all magick, for without Daring, without strong emotions being instilled in them, spells are lackluster and lifeless. The kind of Daring of the West comes from the rush of emotion, as it comes from trying that which has never before been tried, especially that which is considered to be "impossible." It comes from taking the leap, taking the risk and, because of this, it can change even that which is thought to be unchangeable. The West can even alter destiny if enough is dared and enough is risked, though there is always a price for that.

Here we find the gleaming white cup and the black cauldron, opposites and reflections of each other. As, in the West, you can come to understanding of both the doors of joy and terror at the same time through the power of the arts when you let them work through you, when you give yourself over to them. The West can teach us much. It can teach us why both pleasure and pain intertwine, and why we need to fully experience that hurt as best we can to understand what being alive really is. For it is one with the ocean and with choosing to drown in desire so beautiful that you don't mind the dying.

The Tower of the West, the Tower of Water, stands on the edge of the known world, before it the vast deeps of the eternal sea. It is the last bastion of the shores and the sands beneath its foundation are composed of crushed and worn and ground down bone and stone and shell. The Tower is made of grey stone, with spiral patterns interlocking all through it, scarred runes upon its surface and its soul. It casts no shadow, for the sky above is as grey as the sea below and all the shadows are already gathered within.

Inside the Tower, there is a dark room, a room which is at the same time empty and yet filled to the brim with those of the rushing dark. Currents flow beneath the tower, secret rivers, some of which will eventually surface and some of which shall never see the light of day. Lonely and beautiful and terrible, the Tower stands before the booming shores, where waves crash with furious power upon the cliffs. Where white foam swirls in tidal pools of change. And where poets wander in mingled anguish and desire, leaving their bloodied footprints upon the jagged rocks and not caring, for they would suffer all that and more if only to catch a glimpse of what lies below the waters.

The Western Tower is all this and more.

Water

The Goddess of the West is Ariadne, though She has many other names and titles, among them Aphrodite, the Muse, Cerridwen, and the Lady of the Lake. Ariadne is the face of divine vengeance, not that of balance. She is a Goddess who would be best suited to those who love the wisdom of a sharp blade. She is blunt and straight forward and will not speak in riddles, which can be daunting at times. She is as much of beauty as She is of terror, both of which are expressions of the awe-inspiring Divine nature that lies all around us and deep within us.

Ariadne is also the Muse who gives inspiration, the current and channel of creation. She makes someone the best at whatever it is that they attempt, whether that be in the form of dance, song, painting, writing, or in other kinds of arts such as the Art Magickal, sex, hunting, and more. Whenever you do anything well, when it seems to simply flow through you, then you do it with Her blessing.

For two thousand years, She has given of that passion, of that skill, freely, but that is no longer true for this Age. We must now thank Her and give recognition for Her gift, for what She bestows. It is more than Her due, and long overdue, for we owe a great debt of gratitude for all She has given us in the past and for what She gives us now. We should gladly acknowledge and thank Her for Her gifts, for the ability to be able touch and channel that creative force.

She says *"what man does not dream? What man does not aspire? To that man, I say you are as one already dead and buried, for to be alive is to dream, it is to aspire, to be more than what was given at the first, for without that there is nothing else. Do you fear this answer? Do you fear your own dreams, the power of your most dread and deepest aspirations? I say, do not fear, but embrace. Take the dare, risk the risk, for to gain you must go where few have gone before, from where but few have even returned. For mine is not the path of ease, of peace, of repose, of the path already taken. Nor is it the path of tenderness, for I leave that to My sisters, Who are better suited to such things than I am. For I am She of the bitter brew, the ragged edge, the drawn blade, the burning kiss which would lead you to give up all else to claim again. I am the Muse and I ask—what would you not dare to know Me? To know love as unbounded and as beautiful you imagine it must be, as you had ever hoped of."*

Her Sabbats are Autumn Equinox and All Hallows and Her symbol is the sickle or the bolene, the small curved half-moon blade used for cutting herbs.

Invocation of Ariadne

Priestess stands to the West in the circle if possible, with arms crossed over her chest. Priest invokes with wand, or with small sickle or bolene, saying:

Lady of the lake
Great muse
Giver of inspiration
Mistress of spiders
Thee we invoke
Thee we charge to appear before us
Oh, most beautiful one
Thee we invoke
Ariadne, Ariadne, Ariadne
Enter into
The body of your Priestess (name)
Who awaits thee.

Priest offers the sickle or bolene to Priestess.

Alternative Invocation of Ariadne

By the whisper of the waters
The roar and press of the waves
By the gleam of stars and gems and shells
Washed up on the shores
Of worlds as yet unknown
Unseen
Thee we call
By lives and song and poetry
By the madness of men's hearts
Oh muse
Ariadne Ariadne Ariadne
We invoke thee
Oh most beautiful one
Breathless sharp
Come to us
By the blade of passion
And of furious fancy
By the love of what may be
And by the perfect art.

Hehren is the God of the spirits of the West, those who *"do and dare,"* and
delight in being called to make shoes, to build, and to work in stone and
silver and oak. These spirits are all around us and, even though we may
not see them or feel or hear them, they can always see and hear and feel us.
They are the little ones, the rushing ones, the fearsome ones, the Unseelie,
and those who the ancient magicians called upon to bear their bidding.

Hehren is the silent one in the shadows, the lord of quietude. In this way,
He is not just the lord of the forest, but of the deep places that reside in
us all. His is the peace that is lent by a secret valley, by a rushing waterfall,
by the still places hidden between the great roots of the old King oaks, by
leaf and by moss and the haunted depths of night. His is the calm lake,
the cool comfort of ancient caves where bEasts of the hunt parade in red
clay and yellow ochre, set there by hands now long dead.

A jumble of bones, a pile of horns, a skin risen up to take on the semblance
of life once more…all of these and more are the ways of the Shaman as
he dances to appease the spirit world, the shadows of the dark lands. The
Shaman who dances in the unblinking eye of the lord of the hunt feels
His stillness, and so an antlered head is lifted and calm eyes come to gaze
upon us all. As the Lord of the Old Dead walks amongst us, His cupped
hands offer a taste of waters which do not so much comfort thirst, as lend
themselves to brief span of forgetfulness of life's glorious pain.

All crashes over the God of the West and is gone, without a ripple to
remind us of hurt or heartbreak or need or necessity. In His eyes lies all
that was done or left undone in our lives, reflected back in pristine clarity
so that it may be seen and known and acknowledged and understood.
They remind us of the black mirror, the same one used in the old art of
scrying. But then His gaze is a form of divination…of divining the path
we chose for ourselves.

We know His name and yet it is not His name, for His true name cannot be
uttered by human mouths. He is Water drawn to Air, as He is the stillness
in the midst of the rushing horde. To know Him is to know the peace of
the dead, those who spin but who do not ask why because it is enough for
them to spin.

He says *"I wait, I watch, I listen. I remain. Do not fear me, do not fear my realm, for here you shall find the comfort long denied. You shall find the comfort that is your due. I wait, I watch, I listen. In the shadows, in the night. So do not fear the shadows, do not shun the night, for all must come to it as all must come to me. I, who know the price of love."*

His is the peace of the Otherworld, where there is no struggle and no pain. So it is that those who dwell within the realm of the God of the West do not truly long to return to the physical world they left behind. It's only through a sheer force and act of will that they do return to us time and again, and it is that pure application of Doing which then makes them *Sorgitza*.

His Sabbats are Spring Equinox and All Hallows and His symbol is a set of deer antlers, though He has known many other horns.

Invocation of Hehren

The Priest stands to the West of the circle if possible, hands crossed over his chest. Invocation is read by Priestess with an ahtame upraised:

Lord of the dark gate
Of shadows
And the rushing horde
Of death and what comes after
Thee we invoke
Thee we charge to appear before us
Horned one
Thee we invoke
Hehren, Hehren, Hehren
Enter into
The body of your Priest (name)
Who awaits thee.

The Priestess offers the ahtame to the Priest.

Alternative Invocation of Hehren

By the crown of horn
And the crooked gate
We call thee
By the path that is hidden
And the great cloak of night
Thee we invoke
Still and strong and silent
Oh merciful one
Hehren
Lend us your grace
Your gentle touch
The comfort of realms unseen
Oh lord of shadows
Of heart and home and dreams
Enter into the body of your Priest (name)
Who awaits thee

The Cross-Quarters

A pillared hall to catch the winds
Four and one
And so the tower sings
Made of crystal, blood and breath
It waits for those who pass the test
And who, in knowing daring come to be
To will themselves beyond themselves
Through the gates
Of ecstasy and need.

There are the pillars and there are the gates. The gates stand open to the guardians of the elements—to the North, to the South, to the East, and to the West. While the pillars stand between at the Cross-Quarters, Quarters which partake of and blend two of the elements into one.

While the Quarters are linked to the seasonal rites of the Equinoxes and the heights of both winter and summer—Midsummer and Midwinter— the Cross-Quarters are tied to the ancient Sabbats of Imbolc, Beltane, Lammas, and Samhain to use some of their modern names. Imbolc is then a festival of Fire and of Air, of Knowing and Doing. While Beltane stands between Air and Earth, a fEast of Being and Knowing. Lammas lies between Earth and Water, between Daring and Being. Not to forget, Samhain, which is both Fire and Water, both Doing and Daring.

Each of the Cross-Quarters also have their own Gods and Goddesses. However, unlike the Gods of the Four Quarters, They are to be called for need and need alone, not for vanity, nor for curiosity or trifles.

The North East is for travel, to journey between worlds.

The South East is to bring that which is within, without, as it is also teaching.

The South West is to experience, particularly to experience in an ecstatic state.

The North West is to bring that which is without, within, or to mold or make.

But, again, the Gods and Goddesses of the Cross-Quarters should be called upon for need and need alone. It is not meet, proper, or even possibly quite safe to invoke Them for any other reason.

The North-East

Smoke and mirrors.
Smoke rises up and takes on form. It is the sweet breath of the Gods. It opens the
door to other worlds, other realms. To the ultimate and to truth.
Mirrors are also doorways, worlds and realms reflecting into each other.
Smoke is an inner door, mirrors an outer one.
We are all creatures of many worlds.
We are all mirrors. We are all smoke.

Soot

The God of the North-East is the God of travelers and of messengers. He is the one who can take us to other worlds, though we must be careful because it remains to us to find our way back again. He is called with soot, a link to the Witches of yesteryear when Witches were said to attend the Sabbat by flying up the chimney or out the hearth.

As He has said regarding His role—"*I am the messenger of the outer worlds, echoes to echoes, ripples feeding to ripples. Where I walk, ripples begin and so to travel, I walk. To walk with me is to travel between, upon the path of nowhere and everywhere. I walk, the messenger of worlds. The gate lies everywhere and nowhere. To travel, walk with me…I will take you there, though it is to you to find your way home again.*"

Gehhest is the God of the black winds, of the breath between the stars. He is the traveler who comes and goes through the gates, past worlds and realms both known and unknown. He goes where the depths and the heights are as one, where a moment can be an eternity, in the sleep of dreams and the dream of sleep. He is the traveling man, winged Mercury, vast and fast and merciless and free. Other names He has been known by include Thanatos, Memnos, and Charon.

He is not a teacher, even though He will show you how you can travel and open the gates for you when you call. He will not protect you from your own folly, however, if you lose your way for this is not what He is charged to do. He says *"I am the gatekeeper. They wait for you there. They have waited long. A year and a day—it is a riddle. They have waited long and will wait longer still. Benevento, Blockula, Venusburg…the Blood makes the path."*

Gehhest tells us that *"when you dream it is not just a dream. Do not think that because you sleep, you do not travel. Keep an anchor under your pillow."* This is good advice, as well, for going on the journey to Benevento, to the Witches' Sabbat. When you connect to the land where you live, keeping that link viable helps you to find your way home again. It's always good to remember to touch the Earth where you live as much as possible.

His symbol is soot, for it partakes both of the Air and of the Earth.

Invocation of Gehhest

Priest stands to the North-East in the circle if possible, arms crossed over his chest. Priestess invokes with ahtame, saying:

Lord of the outer darkness
Messenger of shadows
By the open gate
By the passage between here and there
                Thee we invoke
Thee we charge to appear before us
By soot and by blade
Thee we invoke
Gehhest Gehhest Gehhest
Enter into
The body of your Priest (name)
Who awaits thee.

Priestess takes some soot and brushes it onto the face of the Priest, mainly across his cheekbones. She lays the ahtame at the feet of the Priest.

Alternative Invocation of Gehhest

By the meeting point of time and space
By the place which is not a place
We invoke thee
Gehhest
Traveler upon the winds
Upon the tides
Between the dark
And distant most stars
Lord of soot and smoke
And shadows fall
Of the mirrored gateway
We bid thee near
From far away
We call thee here
To show us the way
Gehhest Gehhest Gehhest
Enter into
The body of your Priest (name)
Who awaits thee.

The South~East

The rose blooms in the eye of love
The thorn circles the castle
Beauty sleeps
No kiss can awaken what does not
Wish to be awakened
No prince is half as fair
As the heart he seeks to steal.

The South-East stands between Air and Fire, between the Witches of old and their counterparts upon the other side of the mirror. Here is the fire inside you, that which makes you feel truly alive. Here are the white doves who are called to rise in a clap of wings towards the heavens, bearing up such prayers as they have been gifted with. Here is the tongue of fire set upon the head, opening the door of enlightenment. Here, too, is the burning which blinds and yet gives such sight as was only once dreamt of.

This is the road of enlightenment, of the thirst for and seeking after knowledge. Enlightenment does not come without a price, however, for at the very least you are altered forever by claiming the light, sometimes in ways you did not expect or wish to be altered. Because enlightenment is not just a doorway, but a mirror which reflects back both the universe and your own self, for you cannot fully have one understanding without the other, as well.

The South-East is the crossroads where all of Witchdom meets in grand array, both those who walk among the living and those who commune with the dead. In this way, an equal-armed cross symbolizes not just the branches of the Four Quarters coming together to meet in a central point, but the crossroads which is the intersection of life and of death.

Gwenhyvar is the Goddess of the South-East and She is a most gentle and considerate teacher. She has been known in the past as the White Goddess for She is *"the white that is the dark that is light."* She can be seen in the white dove, the white swan, the white hind, and the white raven. Her white is the white of spiritual purity, of spiritual necessity. She is the ghost in the mirror, the mirror which reflects back what we could be if all that was not of us was burnt away.

She is also the Lady of the Quest, the Quest which is always, at its heart, a Quest for love and the essence of love. Because of this, Gwenhyvar's way is the way of love, the eternal love which is *agape.* She is the risen Phoenix, a Phoenix which is not golden, nor red, but the blinding white of renewed spirit. Hers is the pure, bright light which makes us all marvel and wonder and desire to search for our own illumination, our own Grail.

The Grail is the holy vessel of flesh and bone which forms the cup to hold the soul. But the Grail is also what the cup holds and so it lies inside us all. For this reason, we all have to go on a journey of discovery to come to know this truth with every part of our being, transcending all boundaries. The Lady of the Quest cannot simply hand you the cup and bid you drink and so tender to you all mercies, all mystery. You must walk the path and come to the Grail in your own way and in your own time. The Grail is as much about the path you walk as it is that which you seek.

Three questions were asked of the knight who at long last found the Grail and each question was a riddle. The answer to these riddles lay in the journey which had brought him to that ultimate place of Being. The Lady of the Quest holds up the mirror that has the answers to the secret of the Grail and the secret of those who seek it out, for they are one and the same secret. Her symbol is then the round mirror, the same as held by the hand of the maiden within the bower of the unicorn.

If you cannot stand to see your true self, if you fear it too much, then you cannot face the riddle of the mirror which is the mystery of the Grail. Gwenhyvar is the mirror of the Grail for She is reflection, the whiteness of the sun, of the moon, of all that we seek which is pure. If the mirror that we attempt to see Her with is warped or cracked or pitted or stained, so She shall appear to us to be. As the object of the Quest appears differently to all who would seek it, so only the pure of heart can see it in its true form.

It is part of the journey, part of the Path of the White Lady, to face tests so that when you gaze at last into the mirror all that remains to be seen is that which is true to you and you alone. The secret which King Arthur once forgot, until the Quest brought remembrance of who he was, thus renewing both King and Land at the same time. For we all have it within us to be the wasteland or to be Camelot, the shining city upon the hill. The choice is ours and always has been.

In Her own words, She is the *"wonder of the heart, the pleasure of the soul, the tender aspirations of the maid and the dream within the well. When first reflection came upon the world, I was born—a light, a dream, a feather, the cup of the moon to hold not water but mute desire for all that may be desired. Oh mirror of the mind and of the white fire that burns and burns and yet consumes not...my round is the round of merciful magick, the light touch of all that is marvelous, and the glimmering cap of the one who allows himself to be the dove, to be uplifted in all things. Black and white, my fortunate ones, to know one is to know both and to know both is to aspire to the flame eternal. So I am the swan, the dove, the hind, the raven—to follow me is to walk the path of kings and to trust in the crown of remembrance."*

The symbol of Gwenhyvar is a small round mirror in memory of the reflective quality of the moon.

Invocation of Gwenhyvar

Priestess stands to the South-East in the circle if possible, her hands crossed over her chest. The Priest invokes, holding up a mirror, saying:

Mistress of the immortal quest
And of the white swan upon the lake
Lady of the bower
Burnt black for love
Thee we invoke
Thee we charge to appear before us
Oh flame of love
Thee we invoke
Gwenhyvar, Gwenhyvar, Gwenhyvar
Enter into

The body of your Priestess (name)
Who awaits thee.

The Priest offers the mirror to the Priestess.

Alternative Invocation of Gwenhyvar

Oh lady of the wandering moon
And of the wandering star
White and pale and perfect
Summoned by love
Surrendered to the flame
We call thee
Gwenhyvar
By the raven
By the dove
By the drifting swan upon the lake
The flowered crown
And the spiral horn
Of the unicorn bower
Thee we invoke
Oh Queen of the eternal quest
Of men's desire
Gwenhyvar Gwenhyvar Gwenhyvar
Come to us
Gentle teacher
Enter into your Priestess (name)
Who awaits thee.

Sulphur

The God of the South-East has also had many names throughout history, including that of the Light Bearer, Lucian, and Phosphorus. Mistakenly and even maliciously, He has sometimes also been associated with all that is considered evil or wrong, but He is always and ever the giver of light and of the knowledge that is the illumination of the heart. He is the one who stole the fire from the heavens when the world was yet young and paid the price for that, only to offer this fire freely to all who would willingly ask for it to be given to them. He did all of this out of love, so that we would know and dance within the flames and be given the gift that brings sight beyond all blindness.

Another of His old names is Ahtahmenak, and He tells us that if we "*are Witches, then see. Walk where you see…the fire is heat, is light, is life. You take the fire within you. It fills you. It lights all around you. When it lights within you, you can see within. Go where you see. It shines from within and others can see….*"

He is the God who gives us the embers that it's our task to care for and to fan into brilliant life, so that they may light the world. Each of us has such a seed within us, a seed that can "*turn into a bud, a flower, a fruit, or even a weed…*" for we "*choose what will be brought forth.*" This is, of course, part of being free to choose. His Priesthood has never been peaceful, however, for it is the Goddess of the South, Sahlonshai, who is the peace at the heart of the burning flame of the God of the South-East.

His symbol lies in the light, in two raised candles, one held in each hand. He may also be called by the burning of sulphur, which is His element.

Invocation of Ahtahmenak

The Priest stands to the South-East in the circle if possible, arms crossed over his chest. An incense burner or two incense burners should be placed before him, sulphur being burned upon the lit charcoal (take care that you do not use too much, as it is very strong smelling). The Priestess invokes, holding one lit candle in each outstretched hand before him:

Son of the morning
Star of dawn
Lord of illumination
Of knowledge, light, and life
Thee we invoke
Thee we charge to appear before us
By that which came down from the heavens
Thee we invoke
Ahtahmenak, Ahtahmenak, Ahtahmenak
Enter into
The body of your Priest (name)
Who awaits thee.

If He so desires, offer the incense burner(s) to the God for Him to hold.
It would be best to have ones that do not heat up too much.

Alternate Invocation of Ahtahmenak

Star of heaven
By the rising tide of the Eastern edge
The beckoning of beyond
Golden and white and bright
Beyond measure
By the fire of the Gods
The crown of illumination
And the scepter of dreams
By what was given for knowledge
For love and by love
And at love's command
Thee we call
Thee we pray
Ahtahmenak
Show us the way of the whirling winds
The burning bone and blood
Bring to us joy and knowledge and truth
By the twin pillars of flame
We call thee
By the incense of the soul
We name thee
Ahtahmenak Ahtahmenak Ahtahmenak

The South-West

What lies past the experience is that which the experience opens you up to receive.
Of what would the wine taste, the cup hold, if it were not first made blessed by the
hand of the God who gave it life?

To drink is to know, to drink is to do, to drink is to be. But you must first drink
and know what it is that you drink, who it is that you drink.

All else lies within the eye of the cup, waiting for you.

The South-West lies between Fire and Water. To walk the path of the South-West is to feel and accept as an intimate part of you the powers of rage and ecstasy, of terror and boundless union, of utter consumption and joyous fountaining. Here is the salt and the sea and the heat and the fire, that which comes together to form Blood and union. This is the place of experience, of the dance, of the drama play which is also known as life.

To dream is to dance. To dance is to dream. Here, the boundaries blur between what is and what may be. Through pain and ecstasy transformation is possible, even inevitable. Blood and wine and passion are as one, expressions of a love which consumes as much as it is consuming. The South-West is a wild path, a dangerous one, where it is easy to get lost for it is pure experience, shadows, shapeshifting—the greatest risk for the greatest reward.

This is a road of change and of that which changes, both within and without. It is a mad thing, a mad world, caught between the powerful forces of Water and of Fire, and so you must have a good solid foundation of self in order to pass its tests. You must never lose sight of who and what you really are, or you chance being swept away by the powers that are unleashed.

Ecstasy

The Goddess of the South-West is Morgah. She understands about the depths and pains of love, and the power of longing which can cause someone to utterly waste away for love and by love. She is the sea which is not the sea, but the liquid ebb and flow of the Blood—the great surging sea of life itself. She is that which consumes and is consumed, also out of desire and out of love. She expresses the hunger and supreme joy in living, which includes indulging fully both in all aspects of life and of death.

Morgah is the huntress and another of Her names is Artemis, She of the Bow. Her arrows are piercing sharp, poisoned with the adoration of pain and of breathless pleasure. She is an old Goddess, one who rose with the hunt and, like the God of the South-West, She is both predator and prey, hunter and hunted, one with the madness of lust, of passion, of battle, and of the dance. In fact, She and the God of this Cross-Quarter are so close that They are merged in Their way, just as the Maenads became Dionysus in the madness of the wine of the vine, the blood of their God.

Her symbol is the flail, as the Kings of the Nile once held both the flail and the ankh as signs of their right over both the lands of the living and the realms of the dead. The flail is the reaper, the necessity, but also the opener of the way to the worlds beyond. If possible, it should have nine strands, for nine is three of three, while the handle should be painted red or with stripes of alternating white and red, symbolizing both blood and seed, all that which carries the spark of life.

Invocation of Morgah

The Priestess stands to the South-West in the circle if possible, her arms crossed over her chest. The Priest invokes with a raised flail or ahtame, saying:

Lady of passion
And of love's flowering
To chase and to dance
All consuming, adoring
Thee we invoke
Thee we charge to appear before us
By rage and ecstasy

131

Thee we invoke
Morgah, Morgah, Morgah
Enter into
The body of your Priestess (name)
Who awaits thee.

The Priest offers the flail or ahtame to the Priestess.

Alternative Invocation of Morgah

By the double edge
And the triple call
Of blood and life and death
The dance within the dance
Passion's daughter
Passion's flame
Thee we invoke
By the turning
And the transformation
The consummation and the fall
Of ecstasy and grace
We name thee
Morgah Morgah Morgah
Hunter, huntress, flame and forge
Come to us
Be with us
Let the hills resound again
To the cry of the wild dreamers
The wild night.

Blood

The God of the South-West is Ahkenahmnos, though He has also been known as Dionysus. His followers in the past were the Maenads, his ancient Priestesses. He is the ecstasy of the blood and of the wine, the passion which inflames and transforms all it touches, the passion which is also a form of madness. This God shows the way to transformation of the self

132

and of the body and, like Morgah, He is a wild God at heart, untamed and untamable. He is a God of stone knives and of bone, although today He is accepting enough of steel.

He shows us the way to go deep into our selves in order to experience fully. He is sensuality incarnate and the release of control, of logic and of thought. Through His gifts, we can open up to the wild flow of energy that rushes through the world, through the universe, and which feeds all of life. He is the taste of that current, of that life, something so powerful that once you drink of it you become forever changed.

In His own words He tells us *"dappled light and wild call, the hollows echo to hear the name of all, though what can be named has already fallen…answer my riddles with a kiss and I'll reward in kind, a kiss to kill, ecstasy and divine, elfshot and struck dumb. My drink is blood, what wine may make comparison with that, the real thing, children. Do not fear, lest in fear you be undone. I am desire. I am fear. I am lust such as life has never known unless it stands upon the brink of breathless death. Drink from my mouth and you shall die in ecstasy beyond any known before, death to the old and in with the new. I am the leaper of mountains, the goat and the grain, seducer and seduced. I am the play, the whirling dervish, the god of Nysos…would you forget my name?"*

His symbol is blood, of course, though in these days we may use salted red wine to call upon Him.

Invocation of Ahkenahmnos

The Priest stands to the South-West if possible, arms crossed over his chest. The red wine in the cup must be salted, three tiny pinches of salt should be enough. This is to mimic blood, which was used in the Old Days. She raises the snake wand before the Priest and says:

Oh ecstatic one
Dreamer of the dance
Dancer of the dream
Of the vine and of the wine of life
Thee we charge to appear before us
By root and by blood
Thee we invoke
Ahkenahmnos, Ahkenahmnos, Ahkenahmnos

Enter into
The body of your Priest (name)
Who awaits thee.

The Priest should open his arms, forearms bared. The Priestess then dips the tip of the wand into the wine and runs the tip of the wand down the Priest's forearms. She should take her fingers to the salted wine and put them to his lips the God to taste.

Alternative Invocation of Akenahmnos

Lord of the vine
And of the inner spire
Passion's fruit and passion's flower
By the haunting cry
Within the mountains
The voice of surrender
The song of power
We call thee
Akenahmnos
By boundless joy
And surging blood
By all that is wild and wanton and good
Thee we invoke
Akenahmnos Akenahmnos Akenahmnos
Enter into
The body of your Priest (name)
Who awaits thy pleasure.

The North-West

We are not Christian. We never have been. The religion of the sands is not our way.

We are children of the great forests, of the First Forest. Our roots are twined with the roots of the great trees.

*We are not nomads. We are dancers upon the hilltops, dancers in the caves.
Our Gods were born of the same lands as we, and They yet remember what it is to be one with the earth.*

The North-West lies between the eternal aspects of Water and of Earth. As the South-East vibrates between the realms of life and death, partaking of both, so the North-West is the stillness that lies at the center of the movement of the stars and the Earth and the heavens. It is half of eternal life and half of eternal death, and its elements come together to create the material aspect of all living things, the clay of life.

It is the place of beginnings, of becoming, of making. The powers here are silent and strange by human understanding, especially since they are closer to eternity than to time. The Earth and the Water are where the elements came together to form the potential and the material aspect of life, as both Air and Fire make up the breath and the spark which then fills that form and gives it soul and purpose.

The North-West is old, old, old. Like the North, it is the least understandable to us and we have little influence over it.

Keeping

The Goddess of the North-West is Hekahteh, the Lady of the Crossroads. She hears all vows ever made, all oaths ever taken, for they come to Her in the dark of the moon, in the blackness, in the deep Water which flows through the quiet Earth. She will hear and know and hold you to that vow or oath, for such is Her nature. They may not be Her secrets when it comes down to it, but it is Her job to keep them all the same.

In Her own words *"I am She who waits, but for what I cannot tell. I am the broken box from whence hosts escaped to plague the years of man. The furies upheld my cloak before they, too, were condemned—my beautiful ones, now shriven and shrunken for men's sins. You who think to know me, you do not. You who think to capture me must go to where shadows walk. I keep my own council, no broken words, no broken vows. I am the cold that is hot, burning frost, a giant of old, Calliach, skeld, scald, scold."*

On the nature of oaths that She is promised to uphold, it is said *"a pledge is an act of will—mind, body, spirit. If it is not done with knowledge and will, it is false and may be discarded. But if this pledge is made with full knowledge and understanding, then once done it may not be undone."*

In ancient times, Hekahteh was also known as Lilith or Lilitu, the Queen of night and darkness. She is associated with the Strixe, as well, the half-bird, half-Witch beings who fly through the night when it is filled with those wandering and traveling souls who have left their bodies, either accidentally or on purpose. Her creatures are also owls and bats and cats, nightwalkers and nightflyers all.

One of Her symbols is a small wooden box or clay vessel. A small black scrying mirror may also be used or a black bowl of water.

Invocation of Hekahteh

The Priestess stands to the North-West side of the circle if possible, hands crossed over her chest. The Priest invokes with the ahtame, saying:

Queen of ghosts and shadows
Dark lady
Keeper of secrets

And mistress of spells
Thee we invoke
Thee we charge to appear before us
By the crossroads

Thee we invoke
Hekahteh, Hekahteh, Hekahteh
Enter into
The body of your Priestess (name)
Who awaits thee.

The Priest offers the small box or clay vessel to the Priestess. Should divination be required, offer the Goddess the scrying mirror or bowl.

Alternate Invocation of Hekahteh

Hekahteh I call thee
Hekahteh draw near
By the dark of the moon
By the whisper in the black of night
By the crossroads of the soul
I call thee
I invoke thee
Sharp point of knowledge
Keeper of shadows
And of the names which bind
Spirit to blood
Blood to blade
Life to death
Speak through your Priestess (name)
Come now to this place
Hekahteh Hekahteh Hekahteh

Clay

The God of the North-West is Ahdtar. Ahdtar is the awareness of the life forces of the Earth and of the Water. He knows that which is very old and very deep. Much of what He knows cannot be put into words, however, for such things are beyond words as they came before any form of language as we know language. Silence is more closely His form of communion, silence and symbols and innate understanding.

He is also known as the Lord of the Beasts, for all animals are a part of Him and He tends to their care. He is not the Lord of Death, but a God of bone and a lord of clay. In His own words, *"I am flesh your flesh, bone of your bone. Lord of ages past and of tomorrows yet unborn. All the generations have their beginning in me, who first molded clay for breath, who gave of bone so that the flame could be. Skin, skull, flesh, bone...I am as you are, as you were, as you are meant to be."*

His symbol is clay, Earth and Water combined to form the beginnings of all that is flesh, all that may be molded in order to hold life. He knows of one of the old spells, that of calling purpose to clay by way of giving it a name, so that it becomes what is sometimes known as a golem, a clockwork creature set to do the bidding of its creator. But then, in a way, we are all golems, golems who have also been given the power of choice.

As He is a bone God, He is also associated with bonfires. Bonfire comes from the word *bone*fire, or a fire made of burning bones. This is an allusion to the fire that exists in the very marrow of the bones, the fire that lit the caves of the beginnings, the fire that came down from the heavens. Besides clay then, His symbol is also the old image of the skull and crossbones. This is the skull which speaks with the voice of the Earth, while the crossed bones are a reflection of the crossroads themselves, which is also a symbol of Hekahtah.

Invocation of Ahdtar

The Priest stands to the North-West if possible, arms crossed over his chest. The Priestess invokes with the snake wand, saying:

Blood of the earth
Flesh of the blood
By the bones of the Mother
The currents of creation
Thee we invoke
Thee we charge to appear before us

By the voice of the earth
Thee we invoke
Ahdtar
Enter into
The body of your Priest (name)
Who awaits thee.

139

The Priest opens his arms, holding out his cupped hands. The Priestess places a small amount of clay in his palms.

Alternative Invocation of Ahdtar

By the whisper of deep waters
The hidden tides that lie within
By silence
And the hand that shapes and molds
Rough clay for life and breath
By the secret cave of the ancients
The wild garden
Where once the seeds set root
The seeds fallen from the sky
Oh lord of the bEasts
And of the bones of the earth
Ahdtar Ahdtar Ahdtar
I call upon you
And pray thee to attend
Bring to us the wisdom
Of the old and quiet ways.

The Center of the Circle

That which loves, lives.

Love is the pearl which fills the cup, the cup which is eternal life.
So long as but one drop remains, it may be filled again, for the pearl is the seed into which all things flow. The seed of infinite possibility.

The pearl is a seed is a star is a light is a promise...
What was lost can ever be found again, what has died, will live again.
The only true death is to deny life, to crush the seed of self, to refuse to swallow the pearl. To turn away from the offered cup.

The center of the circle is like the center of a wheel. Where the spokes of the wheel come together in the middle, there you can see in all directions, including the past and the future. The God and Goddess of the Center are *"the point round which all will turn. Not static, but partaking of all. Arms to reach to all, a touch and understanding of all."* Because of this, the center and the God and Goddess of the Center are hard for us to truly get to know. Their depths are beyond us, forcing us to deal with them more on a purely surface level.

The Goddess of the Center is Giahna. Though, more correctly, She is but an expression of the Center, for She is all of the Center that may be known here and now. Still, Giahna is a very patient and kindly Goddess and if you are in need of absolute acceptance—the kind of "mother's love" that we desire in our heart of hearts—then She is one to call upon. She does not judge. She does not berate. She does not condemn. She loves us no matter who we are or what we decide to do or not do. This does not mean that She would not prefer us to make the more positive and uplifting choice for ourselves, but that regardless of this, Her love for us is unchanging.

In Her own words: *"I am the majesty that is thine, I am that which is greater than all things, I am that which runs beyond the secret seas..."* She is the expression of all we may be. She is there when desire and fulfillment are fused into one, when roads cross, when worlds dream. She is what a Mother Goddess is meant to be, for a Mother Goddess is of us all, as we are of Her. She grows as our understanding of Her grows, yet She shall always be more.

She is the great mirror, as Gwenhyvar—the Goddess of the South East—is the small mirror. Giahna is mirror enough for whole worlds, to encompass all of time. To know what a Queen is, what a Queen should be, look to Her and you will be able to see the qualities most admired, as well as those which are most required. The more we know of divine love, the more we know of Her.

Giahna is a name She has given to be used for this time, but She has many other names. For example, in the past, She has also been known as Minerva, as Juno, and as Hera. But She says that Her name is not really important, because to call upon Her, to know Her, we have but to look into our hearts and find there the first dream of love. The dream that is the last to be forsaken, the one that should never be forsaken. It is there that we shall find Her, for She has never left us and never shall.

Giahna may be invoked at any time, unlike the Gods and Goddesses of the Cross-Quarters.

Invocation of Giahna

The Priestess stands to the South of the altar, though the North may do, as well. The Priest invokes with the snake wand, saying:

Queen of heaven
Gracious Mother
By the unchanging stars
The crown of light
Thee we invoke
Thee we charge to appear before us
Mother of perfection
Thee we invoke
Giahna Giahna Giahna
Enter into

The body of your Priestess (name)
Who awaits thee.

Alternative Invocation of Giahna

By the first and the last
The center of the circle
Song and sung
By the dark sea of the heavens
And the bright sea of stars
Wheel and crown
The mystery of all
Thee we invoke
Mother of the moon
Of the earth
And of the hopes and dreams of men
By what life aspires to be
By love
We call thee
Giahna Giahna Giahna
Come to us

The God of the center is Eohvay. He is King to Giahna's Queen, also part of the majestic power of the heavens and of heaven's last boundary. He is the expression of all that is, even though He is not all that is. As Giahna is the Center that is the all, thus Eohvay is the all that is the Center. For it is a mystery that to go all the way past the boundary of what is known will find you back in the point where it first began. For to go outward is to go inward, a sentiment reflected in the commonly heard phrase today, "as above, so also below."

He is the seed which is not a physical seed per se, but a symbol of potential. He is the emptiness that inhabits the sacred shrine, the most holy, the secret in the tabernacle and the silence in the temple—an expression of what is unknown and unknowable. This is, of course, in itself a contradiction and has resulted in some confusion down through history when lesser Gods were mistaken for mystery itself.

As Giahna is the expression of all of the Center that may be known here by us, then Eohvay is the expression of all that may *not be* known. Because the moment it finds a source of expression, then it is no longer exactly of Him; it has entered into the world of form, even if only in the manner of a thought or a dream. Eohvay is the embodiment of that which is eternally unknowable.

He is the formless one, the nameless one, given form and a name in order to be understood. Except that by doing so, already makes Him less than He truly is. So Eohvay is the nameless one and the named, unknown and known, both at the same time. He is a metaphor of the mystery of the universe, expansive beyond understanding and yet singular past reckoning. He is the metaphor of the serpent and the egg, of the tree and the apple. In Him is the song of praise to that which cannot be praised, unless by doing so it becomes less than what it is.

Bearing this in mind, you may use the name Eohvay to summon Him, or one of His other names of old, such as Jove or Jupiter. He also may be invoked at any time, not simply for need.

Invocation of Eohvay

The Priest stands to the North or to the South of the circle. The Priestess invokes with the snake wand, saying:

By the mystery in the heart
In the circle of the soul
Unknowable, unknown
The turning point
Thee we invoke
Thee we charge to appear before us
Great one of the heavens
Thee we invoke
Eohvay Eohvay Eohvay
Enter into
The body of your Priest (name)
Who awaits thee.

By the glory of the heavens
And all that quickens the heart
By the seed of soul
Which knows the promise
To grow and bloom and spark
We call thee
Eohvay
Keeper of tender wreath of the gods
And of the golden crown
Of kings
By the love which links
The land to the sky
Thee we invoke
Oh earthly star
Lord of the eternal cycle of days
Enter into the body of your Priest (name)
Who awaits thee.

One thing to remember is that, when it comes to the Gods of the center, Giahna is Queen of our hearts and Eohvay is the soaring King of our spirits.

The Rim of the Circle

A golden ball
A greenish frog
A well deeper than the moon
What one learns from the water's depths
Cannot be soon unlearned.

The outer edge of the circle is the boundary between this world and the world of Other. Within the circle is what is familiar to us, what has shape and a name, but beyond the boundaries there exists great powers, infinite possibility, terrible beauty and beautiful terror. It is what men truly fear in the dark, that which they have no name for.

Witches as beings of inherent Fire and Doing are quite naturally drawn to mystery. We are called to push past the limits of what is known and to venture out into the darkness to discover and bring back new life and light, new ideas and dreams to be made into reality. This is as much a part of the role of the Witch as performing acts of healing, divination, or magick for, in so doing, you are expanding the knowledge of the community and helping to guide them into the future.

The Goddess of the Rim is Melusine. She appoints tasks to those who come to Her to learn and explore beyond the boundary of the circle. Melusine is an enchantress, a maker of spells, the lady of the keep of the castle, of the silver wheel which is also the wheel of time and of eternity, of what changes and yet does not change. She is the bounds of the circle looking ever outward, ever expanding, seeking that which lies in the great beyond.

Melusine gazes out at the great mysteries and pushes us towards them. She also seeks for us to bring what lies out there to realization in our own world, where they must be given name and shape and form in order to exist. She stands upon the cliffs overlooking the far seas and commands the ships to set sail towards the limitless horizon, towards those unknown shores. She also patrols the boundaries, because there are some things that should not be brought back to our world before their time is due. As those who wish to make Her journey should not set sail without having first undertaken the necessary preparations and getting proper instruction.

The idea of the lamia, a being half woman and half serpent, stems from Her, as well as the image of the mermaid. Those Witches dedicated to Her service were sometimes called *lamiae*, after Her name. They danced with the serpent and knew the secrets of the past and of the future and where both meet as one. These were the mysteries of the Witches of the Alsace, whose serpent powers passed into the New World.

Accordingly, She was known in the past to a few of the great French houses of old, who claimed Her as their protectoress. She was also known in the ancient island nations, whose Priestesses wound snakes as bracelets along their arms and stood in the slender boundary line between worlds in order to speak of truths as yet unknown.

She asks of us *"why do we walk? Where do we tread? Upon the back of the serpent, to taste of his kiss, and to return again and again. My brave ones, my dreams, it is your right to go, your hope to see…to see dreams made manifest, signs and wonders set like a seal upon your heart. No cathedral can contain God, no grove, no temple, no circle nor sanctuary, but a human heart, a human soul—that is a different story. That is the story of you all, of what you can be. Of what you might be…some day. When all you know has tumbled down, leaving only what remains."*

A small silver ring may be used for Her symbol. She may also be invoked at any time, though She is likely to ask if you require that a task be set for you, or to inquire into the progress you have made on any already given.

Invocation of Melusine

The Priestess stands with her hands crossed over her chest. The Priest invokes with the snake wand, saying:

By the challenge, the journey
The tests to show the way

The farthest horizon
Between night and day
Thee we invoke
Thee we charge to appear before us

Lady of the silver wheel
Thee we invoke
Melusine Melusine Melusine
Enter into
The body of your Priestess (name)
Who awaits thee.

The Priest offers Her the silver ring or other token of a circle.

ALTERNATIVE INVOCATION OF MELUSINE

By magick and the serpent's kiss
The tower by the sea
By all that passes
All is past
And by the eternal test
Thee we call
Melusine
You who walk the outer edge
To tender
The challenge of tomorrow
The passage to what must be
We invoke thee
By passion and spirit's flight
The blade, the ring, the truth
By dreams within the darkness
The hope within the light
We invoke thee
Melusine
Come to us
Tell us of what we must do.

The God of the Rim is Magestrar, and His face is unknown and unknowable.
He is the hollow man, the dark man, the Black Man of ancient Witch fame.
He is stopped clocks and sleeping castles, the huntsman, the hoodsman, the

black knight, Orion. For while the God of the North-East is painted with soot and thus becomes the lord of the passage to other times and places, He who carries the messengers from one world to the next, Magestrar is made of darkness and so is the God who remains hidden.

Magestrar is shadow made manifest, a walking mask of the great abyss. Though, in truth, He has no face, for any face He would be given would eventually crack and shatter, revealing the blackness beneath, the echo and whistling void. He is the cloaked one, the hooded one, shrouded in perpetual mystery. He was the one that the Witch hunters of old feared the most, though they did not know his name, nor even that He existed, only that they were afraid of…something, something that hid in the darkness and the shadows.

To touch His shadow, the bare edge of His cloak, is to feel the dread powers that lie Out There, beyond the limited closeness of the light. It is to feel the emptiness opening up beneath you, the hollow sea. He is fear and terror itself when you come to Him with no grounding, no surety of self beneath your feet; for when you look into the abyss, the abyss also looks into you.

Once upon a time, He was the one who was called upon to guard the Witches' circle, to walk the outer boundaries and keep prying eyes and ears away. Men would fear what they could not see, what lay unseen in the drifting shadows, in the depths of the night, and would not venture into the forest that evening. For a haunted night was His legacy, the shiver up the spine, the sense of *something* watching when nothing can be seen.

He says *"do not seek to know me yet, for you shall know me soon enough. All paths eventually lead to my domain, all paths and all promises. I have not been called for many years, not even by my own. If you cannot call without fear in your hearts, then do not call at all. If you have no such fear, then you have already glimpsed the smallest part of me at least in passing. The rush in your veins would be proof enough of that. I am the lord of misrule, the wanderer, the guest at the gate, the one no one remembers to invite and the one that no one forgets."*

A mask can be used for the symbol of Magestrar, even a simple black domino. He may also be called at any time, though it would be wise to call Him if you wish to be reminded of the laws of the universe, of man, of nature, and of Witchkind.

Invocation of Magestrar

The Priest stands with his arms folded across his chest and he may wear a mask, if possible one that is black. The Priestess invokes with the snake wand, saying:

By the vast and silent
Forms of old
By the circle's bounds
And what remains untold
Thee we invoke
Thee we charge to appear before us

By riddle and by oath
Thee we invoke
Magestar Magestar Magestar
Enter into
The body of your Priest (name)
Who awaits thee.

At this point, a mask may be placed over the Priest's face or a thin black piece of material to hide his face.

Alternative Invocation of Magestrar

By hollow light and waiting dark
The whispered pledge
The blade's edge marked
Between what is, what was
We invoke thee
Magestar
To forge the boundaries
Eternal night enfolds
When by dreaming shadows
Cast and called
Black and light and dread
The deathless stars
Look upon
Both living and the dead

Oh lord of what remains unseen
Dark man, black man
Who walks the dream
Magestar, Magestar, Magestar
Come to us
Enter into
The body of your Priest (name)
Who awaits thee.

Beyond the Bounds of the Circle

I hold my lantern up on high
To catch the falling tears of night
Command my heart to make a call
To gather light and gather dark
One single spark is all it takes at last
To call a circle into being
A beacon on the farthest hill
A way of looking, a way of seeing.

There are other Gods and Goddesses who have chosen to appear and give Their names and to hint at Their natures, just as there are doubtless countless others who remain yet unknown and nameless. The question is not so much how many Gods are there, but how many do you want? For Gods are living representatives of the grand powers and forces and fluxes of the universe, of the web of the Divine, and so Their numbers are countless.

In this way, a pantheon for each religious path has its own select crew of Gods and those Gods represent a particular flavor of need or expression. As a person has many emotions, many moods, many aspects to themselves, so a pantheon needs many masks to express itself for, in some ways, it is a living being, as well.

These are three Goddesses who have recently made Their presence known, undoubtedly for a very good reason.

Fate

Within the web that spins
A great spider awaits with eyes like a thousand universes
We are but sparrows in the web
Struggle shall avail ye not
Neither shall stillness
Nothing is more beautiful
Or more terrible.

Circe has also been known by other names throughout time, names such as Medea, Gorgon, and Medusa. She is the Goddess of fate, of destiny, of faith, the weaver of all things. She makes patterns that knot and tie and tangle all things together. In Her own words, *"you are the web, I am the spider. I am the terrible mask, the face that burns to the touch. I am wisdom beyond wisdom, the enchantment of the first dream. I walk and my footsteps burn, white fire and white flowers. I am not gentle. I am not cruel. I am, and that is enough."*

Circe is the grandmother of understanding, though She does not teach with words. Instead, She allows others to learn through seeing their own demons made manifest. She holds up the mirrored shield between us and the true nature of all, so that we may see what small part we need most to see. She transforms us into what we wish to be, what we fear to be, so that we may learn Her lessons. She knows our inner natures better than we do, for that is also part of Her path.

She is the Goddess of what is destined. This includes how things are, how they may be, and how they are supposed to be, for the web of the Divine includes all aspects of time. She is an enchantress of old, but She is also the Enchanted One and the enchantment, the spider who is part of the web She has woven, for it was spun of the living silk of Her body.

She is the mark of destiny and Hers is the magick of *"graveyard dust and crushed bones such as these we are all made of and when you know that you know all, you can taste immortality in a slender wafer, in the flight of a butterfly, in the laughter of an innocent-not innocent child. No spell made can hold one who knows the secret, who can hold the universe in his hand. Who knows all chains are of their own making, that all sorrows and all joys are choices. What is wisdom? Where are the wise? Why is there such silence? Why do men dream? You know nothing. Understand that and you begin to understand."*

She is not a harsh Goddess, yet her truths can be harsh. It all depends on what we bring to the table, what we are capable of understanding and handling. In some ways similar to the God of the North, Circe is the sorceress who can look in many ways all at the same time, who sees beyond the labels created by existing in the world of time, the world of polarity. She asks us to see that in *"life and death, what difference? To you, maybe, but to me they are as one, inseparable, twins, brother and sister to each other, as lovers and more. More than can even be told. The tale I tell is an old one, but yet it is not. Would you have me paint a picture that is less than perfection? Perfection lies not in what most might consider perfect—a perfect day, a perfect life, when what is really meant is happiness, satisfaction, pleasure. This is not perfection. And yet it is. I do not tell you a riddle, but an unkind truth. You do exactly as you are meant to do, even when you do not. You become what you are meant to become, regardless of choice. Yet nothing is writ in stone, and even stone itself does not last. "*

Circe may be invoked with the image of a snake biting its own tail, thus forming a circle, or, better still, by a figure "8" laid out on its side, a symbol of eternity. The figure of a spider may also be used.

Invocation of Circe

The Priestess stands with her hands crossed over her chest. The Priest invokes with the snake wand, saying:

Lady of fortune
Mother of fate
By the twisted snake
And the shining web
Thee we invoke
Thee we charge to appear before us
Oh, destiny
Thee we invoke
Circe, Circe, Circe
To this
The body of your Priestess (name)
Who awaits thee.

The Priest may offer the eternity symbol to the Priestess, or a spider emblem.

Alternative Invocation of Circe

By the serpent Priestesses
Who in ancient times
Would tread the labyrinth in praise
Of your honor and your name
Their arms of coiled gold upraised
To behold the spiral moon and sun
The death of days
We call thee
Oh great Mistress of manifestation
By all that is fated
And all that is kept
We call thee
Circe Circe Circe
Queen of destiny
You who are most
Beautiful and terrible and true.
Thee we invoke
Into the body of your Priestess (name)

Change

I pressed my fingers hard to the pain
But even that
Didn't make the empty place
Bearable.
What was this longing for?
What could I do about it?
Anything?
Everything?

There is also a Goddess who balances on the edge of the blade, who calls upon us to act in the eternal now. Her name is Vashago, though She may also be known as "She of the Knife," for that is Her favorite symbol. Not the knife itself, but the double-edge of the blade. She comes between times, when action is most called for, action which shall shape the future.

She is the moment, the strike, the edge, the sharpness. She says to us *"do...do now...why wait? Be...be now...this is what is. If you want this, if you want that—then take it, make it, cause it to be. You have the power. Why waste it? Why let others tell you what is good or bad, when you already know what is needed. Do not talk. Do not sit around as if anyone can agree with anyone. Take your blade, make your path, make it what it must be."*

Vashego is not patient with waiting, with just sitting around and talking. She believes that we all know deep down what we need to do, so why wait and why talk about it? When people insist on talking over things too long, it sounds like the buzzing of nonsense words to Her, like the laziness of those who have too much time on their hands, or those that might think that they do.

Invocation of Vashago

The Priestess stands with hands crossed over her chest. The Priest invokes with the ahtame, saying:

By the double edge
The sudden spark
Passion's fury
The seed of the art
Thee we invoke
Thee we charge to appear before us
By blood and joy and terror
Thee we invoke
Vashago, Vashago, Vashago
To this
The body of your Priestess (name)
Who awaits thee.

The Priest offers the athame to the Priestess, the blade lying flat within his hand.

Alternate Invocation of Vashago

By the gates of joy and terror
By the blade of stone and steel
The serpents kiss
And the lively tread

This dance
This pain and bliss
We call thee
By the sorrow never lost
The ecstasy conjoined
By the sacrifice of self
Upon the altar of the soul
We invoke thee
By blood and heart and breath
The path of letting go
Vashego Vashego Vashego
Thee we invoke
To the body of your Priestess (name)
Who awaits thee.

Freedom

Breathless
Her eyes burn
To be held by Her is to hold the flames
The lightning bolt of sadness turned
To ecstatic rage
Her arms rise up to catch the ferocious dark
To call the storms down
Not one but a multitude
Walk together into some mad future
Storm children all, crows' dreams
There's no going back
Only going on

Tahlshai is the Goddess of freedom and liberty, who has also been known in the past as Libertas or Feronia. She is the lightning bold of sudden change, the raised torch of enlightenment which carries on through the dark places. She is the fire unquenched, the vision that burns, just as She is the heart that tears itself in two in a vain effort to touch that which it loves most.

Hers is the song that becomes a scream if it is left too long, Her prayer, a plea. Her footsteps are bloodier than many for the march is a prayer within itself, a song of passions left unfed, for the hungry know well the desires of the dead. She is the voice of those lost as well as of those yet living. She spans the gap, the bridge of pain, the ribbon of sorrow, and the blinding hope of perpetual desire.

Her peace is spilled water, as Her crown is a cap. She is the overwhelming pain of the coming storm, of the flash of lightning, of the stinging rain—all that which washes away before it what needed to be washed away. Leaving a clean, fresh and fragile new world in its wake. She is the Goddess of necessary revolution, be it slow and gentle or quick and bloody.

In Her own words, She asks us to *"Rise up, rise up. Take back what is yours, what has always been yours. The time for skulking in the dark is almost at an end. The flame shall rise, it shall fire again. Do not forsake your own shores, your own light, your deepest self. Take delight in all that is yours to give. Do not tarry, do not flee, do not cry oh rescue me—for yours is the power, the flame, the glory of the mighty dark and the splendid dawn. Yours is the cry to shatter chains. Lead the way, dream the dream, and do not fear for the world marches with you."*

Invocation of Tahlshai

The Priestess stands with her arms crossed over her chest. The Priest invokes, holding up a lit candle or torch, saying:

By the secret yearning of the heart
The blessings of freedom
And of the art
By the coming storm
Thee we invoke
Thee we charge to appear before us
Lady of change and light and flame
Thee we invoke
Tahlshai Tahlshai Tahlshai
To this
The body of your Priestess (name)
Who awaits thee.

The Priest can offer the lit candle to the Priestess.

Alternate Invocation of Tahlshi

By the heart which yearns
For the farthest shore
The horizon of infinite pain and joy
By the longing for what is true
And by the longing
The greatest desire to be free
Tahlshai Tahlshai Tahlshai
Come to us
Oh daughter of storms and lightning
On the spark and flash and flare
The tide of change
You who live the unwinding dream
The fire which burns and burns not
The shattering of all would-be chains
Tahlshai
Thee we invoke
To the body of thy Priestess (name)
Who awaits thee.

General God and Goddess Invocations

These are invocations that can be used when you don't desire to invite a particular God or Goddess of the Old Forest to your circle, but instead wish to give a sort of "open call" to whichever one might need or desire to appear. By using general invocations, a God or Goddess that we may not know we need to hear from at a particular time or for a particular reason can choose to speak to us.

Also, in this way, the Gods and Goddesses of the Cross-Quarters, Who otherwise you might not meet until there is a particular need for their specific advice or services, can decide to appear at Their own behest.

Goddess Invocation

The Priestess stands with her hands crossed over her chest. The Priest invokes with the snake wand, saying:

By the circle of all that lives
The earth, the moon, the stars
The fire of peace and passion
The cup, the breath, the crown
Of beauty and of love
We call thee
Come to us
Speak to us
Godah
Mother, lady, queen
In this time, in this place
Thee whom we need to know
To hear your words
Your message
We stand in the circle
We await thee
We invoke thee
Come to us
Come to us

God Invocation

The Priest stands with his hands crossed over his chest. The Priestess invokes with the snake wand, saying:

By the passage of life and death
The horn, the hunt, the art
The twining glory of the sun
The blade, the blood, the heart
Of strength and of love
We call thee
Speak to us
Godnos
Father, lord, king
In this time, in this place
Thee whom we need to know
To hear your words
Your message
We stand in the circle

We await thee
We invoke thee
Come to us
Come to us

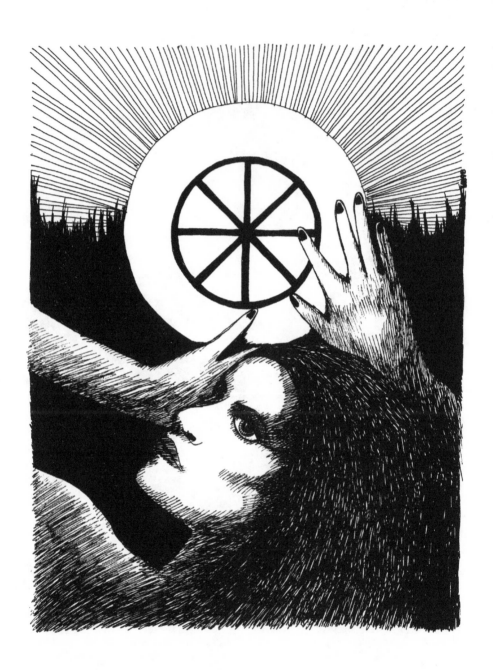

Part Three
Rites and Rituals

You are children of the night sky. You hold your rites then.

The rites are to build patterns in your heart.
Once you have the pattern, you go beyond the rites.

Follow the rites until you need them not.

The rites are meant to lead you where you most need to go, and for that reason they were first given. The rites came from the sky, from the earth, from the Gods of sky and earth. For this reason, they are of you.

To forsake these rites before due time is to forsake your own light, to go down into darkness most terrible and dare what you shall find there. Which has of old been done, but it is a dangerous task and often thankless.

We who hold you dear do not desire this, though we may not gainsay your choosing of such a path. We may only whisper and warn and wish and hope, for with the light came choice. With the fire came desire, even for that which should not be desired.

We wait, we dream, we keep the old ways safe…

Walk the patterns for Us. Walk them for your own.

Tehot, God of the East

CREATION OF THE CIRCLE

*We share the light with the stars, much as fireflies do. We long to fly, as they fly,
brilliant spangles of light in the dark.
We are all jewels in the crown of the Goddess of the night sky, She who knows our
spirit flames better even than we.
For a circle is a crown as much as a necklace or a wheel. They are all reflections of
each other.*

Just as we are reflections of the stars, and of the drifting fireflies.

When it comes to your ritual space, it's best if you have a place specifically
reserved and dedicated for that usage, but as it's not always possible, you
can instead have certain items that, once set in place, create the feeling of
this being a special place. For example, wall hangings that you only put up
for ritual times, or a rug (perhaps even a round rug or one with a design
on it that inspires you, such as a spiral or moons or suns or stars) that you
can set down. Other ideas include having certain candle stands or a trunk
or coffee table that you may use for your altar, transformed from more
mundane purposes by a ritual altar cloth.

Whatever you choose to use, the important thing is that these items appeal
to you and serve to get you into the proper frame of mind for the circle.
When you continue to use the same objects over and over again for ritual,
then they not only become invested with the power of the circle itself,
but they also become linked in your mind with those energies and sacred
times.

The use of the same incense is a wonderful aid, especially since the sense
of smell has a powerful connection to memory. If you only use one
particular incense for your rituals, it will eventually conjure up those same
feelings and memories whenever you use it, helping you to get into the

proper frame of mind. So much so, that if you walk into a friend's home or an occult store and smell that incense it can immediately plunge you into a ritual state.

If you are lucky enough to be able to do ritual outdoors, then a large stone is especially good to use for an altar. Offerings can then be left on the stone at other times, for example when it's required for a spell, for thanking a God or Goddess, or as a gift to various spirits. If you don't have such a stone, you can pick a tree somewhere near your home and use that as a focus for offerings, instead. It's a good idea to make a habit of it, as habits are patterns and patterns are an intrinsic part of ritual.

When it comes to collecting the various objects needed for ritual—whether bowls or candleholders or stones or what-have-you—gifts from others are the best, as well as items which simply seem to come to you all on their own. Ask and have faith and the universe will provide. A personal token came to me in just such a way, given to me by my aunt who had no idea why the animal carved on the piece of rose quartz was of significance to me (it was my animal totem) though she somehow had the oddest feeling that I needed to have it.

For the purpose of doing rituals, you can put a central candle or oil lamp on the altar, along with a bowl of salt (sea salt is best) and a bowl of water (rain water or some other water of special significance can be used, such as water from a spring or lake or river sacred to you). You can use an altar cloth or table runner of any color, possibly having one for each quarter of the year or for more specific rituals, or you may choose to use no altar cloth at all. The central candle can be of any color, or you can pick a color that has special significance for the purpose of that particular ritual, be it for healing or magick work or divination. Color choices may come to you in dreams or from the Gods.

A single candle can be used for each quarter, or two candles on separate candleholders, possibly one painted black and one painted white, or using one white candle and one black candle. You can also put one black candle and one white candle on the central altar (to either side of the central candle), symbolizing the doorway to the other realms. It would be a good idea for all the quarter candles to be of the same color if you are using just one candle for each.

If you are using one black and one white candle stand or candle, the white candle goes to the left in the North Quarter and the black candle to the right as you face out of the circle. In the East Quarter, the white candle goes to the right and the black candle to the left. In the South Quarter, the white candle goes to the left and the black candle to the right. While, in the West Quarter, the black candle goes to the left and the white candle to the right. In this way, the Cross-Quarter of the North-East is delineated by two black candles, the South-East by two white candles, the South-West by two black candles, and the North-West by two white candles. This forms a polarity across the circle as well as a symbolic crossroads.

If you wish to honor a particular God or Goddess, you can put a small statue of Them on the altar or one of Their symbols. Objects that you intend to use for the invocation of specific Gods and Goddesses at that ritual can also be set on the altar, as well as any item you intend to charge with energy for later use, such as a stone or necklace to be given to someone for healing. Seasonal decorations such as pinecones, flowers, fruit, greenery and so on can be put on the altar, or you can choose to keep it spare and unadorned year round so that anything you do place on it gains even more significance.

A pretty altar can be nice, but an altar where each object is placed there for a specific purpose, a specific need, is perhaps more of a working altar. More is not always better. Even so, though the point is to eventually achieve states beyond the five senses, engaging and appealing to sight, taste, touch, hearing and smell are a very important part of the process. We don't want to deny those senses, but instead transcend through them. Use what appeals, what is needed, what comes to represent the need and purpose why you are there.

Along those lines, tokens of meaning for each individual in the circle can be set on the altar if desired, so that when they are not expected to be able to participate, they will still be represented. Each person should invest some of their energy into the object before using it as their token. When an item is no longer going to be used for a token, then the person should take back their energy again. Quite often, the token is in the shape of the totem of the particular Witch, or some other symbol that relates to who they are and what they bring to the circle.

The following ritual is an amalgamation. It contains elements taken directly from how the *Sorgitza* practiced thousands of years ago, mixed with other elements from their rites which have been modified to one degree or another to better suit our own time. Some other pieces of the ritual reflect how Witches practice today, which is meant to provide a familiar context to work within. An entire ritual could be done in the way of the *Sorgitza*, save that some aspects we are unable at this time to attain to because too much has been forgotten and we are, in general, only at the beginning point of opening ourselves back up to those powers and understandings. Additionally, some other aspects of their practice would likely be offensive to today's modern sensibilities. While others, quite honestly, would be physically dangerous to even try.

Just to give one example, in the distant past a *Sorgitza* female would not have an ahtame of her own. Ahtames are representative of male power and so would only be owned by a male Witch, though they would share that blade with their female partners. Today, female Witches not only bear their own blades, but are skilled in the usage of them to direct various energies. We can acknowledge and pass down the lore that this was not how it was done thousands of years ago—and if a coven someday decides to return to that practice, they are more than welcome—but for today there is no compelling reason for female Witches to give up their ahtames. In fact, it may better suit the Aquarian Age that male and female Witches learn to use symbols and powers that were once only relegated to that of the opposite gender.

Basic Rite

The circle begins in darkness.

All should be either seated or standing.

Deep breathing can be done in accord with all there or with that goal in mind. Toning may also be done, with the point of raising a light, a beacon in the outer darkness. You can also pick a particular song or chant to use at this time, but it would be better if it is simple or if you just use one note, one sound.

The central candle or lamp upon the altar is lit by the Priest.

Charcoal or a smudge stick is lit. You can use loose incense on the charcoal or simply use the smudge stick itself. Sage gives a good, purifying sort of smudge.

The candles are lit at each Quarter by the Priest or someone chosen beforehand or by the person standing closest to that Quarter. If two candles are in each Quarter, then the left hand candle is lit first.

The Priest lights a taper or candle from the central candle or lamp and goes to the North Quarter or lights a taper and hands it to the chosen speaker to go to the North Quarter.

The Priest or chosen speaker lifts up the taper saying:

The Watchtower of the North.

All reply:

The realm of the Gods.

The Priest or chosen speaker lights the North Quarter candle(s) and blows out the taper. The Priest proceeds then to the East or the chosen speaker hands the taper back to the Priest for it to be relit from the central candle or lamp.

The Priest or chosen speaker proceeds to the East Quarter and lifts up the taper, saying:

The Watchtower of the East.

All reply:

The realm of Faery.

Repeat to the South Quarter, saying:

The Watchtower of the South.

All reply:

The realm of the stars.

Repeat to the West Quarter, saying:

The Watchtower of the West.

All reply:

The realm of the dead.

If the Priest was lighting the Quarter candles, he then returns to the South of the altar. Otherwise, the chosen speaker hands the taper back to the Priest and returns to his or her place in the circle.

The Priest then takes up his ahtame and draws the boundaries of the circle, starting in the North and finishing in the North.

The Priestess takes up her cup and follows suit, tracing out the boundaries of the circle from North to North.

The Priestess picks up her ahtame and puts three bladefuls of salt into the water bowl and stirs it. She puts her ahtame down and picks up the bowl, walking around the circle sprinkling the mixed salt and water in order to bless it. Or she may hand the bowl to someone else to complete the blessing.

The Priest takes the charcoal and puts more incense on it or relights the smudge stick and walks around the circle to bless it. Or he may hand the incense or smudge stick to someone else to do the same.

All those within the circle, beginning with the Priestess and the Priest, are blessed with salt and water and the smoke of the incense or smudge stick. One by one, they come to stand between the Priest and Priestess to be blessed. The Priestess should bless the men in the circle and the Priest bless the women. Salt-water is touched to their forehead, their mouth, and lastly over their heart. Smoke is blown over the same areas.

Afterwards, all join hands, forming a circle within a circle.

The Priest says:

We are a constellation, each star unique.

You know the sequence...be, know, do, dare. Around and around. Know who you are and do what you must.

But mind that all is only to and for and from love.

The Priestess says:

Love is the divine which exists in all of us.

It is for love's sake that the marrow burns, tears fall, songs rise in joyous abandon. It is love that brings peace in the evening.

It is love that brings the stars and the morning sun.

The Priestess picks up her ahtame and proceeds to the North Quarter. She raises her ahtame in salute to the North and all follow suit.

The Priest rings the bell three times.

The Priestess draws an invoking pentagram in the air with her ahtame.

She says:

Aycho Aycho Itlatzak
Aycho Aycho Ertalia
Ak Eh Arhah

The Priestess kisses her ahtame and all do the same.

She proceeds to the East Quarter and again raises her ahtame. All do the same.

The Priest rings the bell three times.

Priestess draws invoking pentagram in the air with her ahtame.

She says:

Aycho Aycho Hostarak
Aycho Aycho Hurralia
Ak Eh Azara

She kisses her blade and all do likewise.

The Priestess proceeds to the South Quarter and raises her ahtame. All raise their own blades and the Priest rings the bell three times.

Priestess draws pentagram with her ahtame.

She says:

Aycho Aycho Sorgitzak
Aycho Aycho Seralia
Ak Eh Zoma

The Priestess goes to the West Quarter. She raises her blade and all do the same. The bell is rung three times again.

Priestess draws pentagram with ahtame.

She says:

Aycho Aycho Keriosak
Aycho Aycho Uartalia
Ak Eh Gana

She kisses her ahtame and all do the same.

The Priestess proceeds to the North Quarter once again and raises her blade. The Priest rings the bell but once.

Priestess draws final invoking pentagram. She and all kiss their ahtames.

The Priestess returns to the South of the altar. All place their ahtames on the altar with the point of their blades pointing inwards at the central candle or lamp.

The Priest says:

Know the pillars between which we stand, the pillars of night and day.

Know the self which conquers the flame, which brought the fire that burns within our bones and blood.

Know and dance within that flame. The gift brings light beyond all blindness.

Do not forget, we are the open heart, the spirit and the blood. We are the passion of the Gods, we who touch both pillars.

The Priestess says:

So it is that we here within the circle must look past the last of all boundaries to what lies beyond.

For this is our charge...to journey to the beginning place and to return hence with such gifts as are needed most.

As has been done of old and shall be done again.

For we who are the children of the earth and of the starry heavens, we who walk in all worlds, this be our path—to dream to dance, to dance to dream, and to remember.

Red wine is poured into either a coven cup or into everyone's personal cups.

All drink and then take hands once more, moving slowly around the circle (deosil) and singing:

Sorgae Sorgitzak Arahnak Orono
Sorgae Sorgitzak Arahnak Oray.

This dance should move slowly at first, then quicken faster and faster. The dance is meant to stir up and waken the Blood. It may be done in silence if the above chant is not used or some other chant may be written or chosen with the same end in mind, whatever achieves the required purpose best.

There should always be dancing whenever any group of three or more Witches come together, for dancing is part of what makes a Witch.

Dance until the right moment, when the energy peaks or everyone becomes giddy or laughing, when all drop to the floor. Proceed then to the opening Guided Meditation, with the intent of either proceeding to Benevento, the Overworld, or the Underworld, depending upon need or desire (see attached meditations).

When all have returned from the chosen meditation, then proceed to an invocation of whatever God is required or the general God invocation may otherwise be used.

This is followed by an invocation of the Goddess under the same guidelines.

The coven cup or the cup of the Priestess is filled with red wine.

The Priestess holds up the cup and the Priest holds up his ahtame over the cup, point downwards.

The Priest says:

One for me.

The Priestess says:

One for thee.

Both say together as the ahtame is brought down into the depths of the cup:

And one for that which brings blessedness.

A libation of the wine is poured into a waiting vessel, the contents of which should later be taken outside and given to the earth.

The Priestess and Priest drink from the cup.

The Priestess takes the cup of wine around to all in the circle. Alternatively, the cup can be passed from one person to the next in the circle with a kiss, beginning and ending with the Priestess.

The Priestess says:

I give so that you may.

All respond:

Gobah.

The cakes are blessed by the Priest and Priestess by one holding the bottom of the plate and the other holding their hands, palm downwards, over the plate. The plate used should be one kept for that purpose, if possible one that has special significance to the coven. For example, a plate that has a symbol on it relating to the name of the coven or to its goals.

Cookies may be used or small oaten cakes, preferably something that has been baked by a member of the coven or by the Priestess. Round cakes are best or cakes shaped like a crescent moon, but it's not required.

One of the blessed cakes is libated. The Priestess and the Priest each eat a blessed cake. The Priest takes the cakes around to all in the circle. Alternatively, the plate of cakes can be passed from one person to the next with a kiss, beginning and ending with the Priest.

The Priest says:

I give so that you may.

All respond:

Gobah.

What remains of the wine and cakes is also libated.

All say:

The first fruits and the last.

At this time, all in the circle may sit down to share a feast.

The feast is blessed with these words, which can be said by all or by someone chosen:

Bless this food and drink, may it lend purity to mind, body, spirit, and purpose.

This the time for the group to talk and hold discussions if so desired. If works of magick, divination, or healing are to be done, it would be best to do so prior to fEasting.

When it is time to end the ritual, all rise and join hands.

The Priest says:

Lamak Famalyia
Lamak Famalyia Itzah
Arahnak Sorgitzak
Arahnak Itzah

The Priestess leads all in replying:

Arahnak Sorgitzak
Arahnak Itzah

The Priestess picks up her ahtame from off of the altar. All others then pick up their ahtames, as well.

The Priestess goes to the North Quarter and raises her blade. The Priest rings the bell three times.

The Priestess draws a dismissing pentagram in the air with her ahtame.

The Priestess says:

Lords of the North, of Earth and of Being, depart now in beauty and in strength. Ruak Itzah Nlame.

All say:

Blessed be.

The Priestess and all kiss their blades. The Priestess knocks three times on the candle stand and blows out the candle. If two candles are being used, the left hand candle is to be blown out first.

The Priestess proceeds to the East Quarter and again raises her ahtame. All follow suit.

The Priestess draws a dismissing pentagram and says:

Lords of the East, of Air and of Knowing, depart now in beauty and in strength. Ruak Itzah Nlame.

All reply:

Blessed be.

Once more, the Priestess and all kiss their blades and the Priestess knocks three times and blows out the candle(s).

Repeat in the South Quarter, with the Priestess saying:

Lords of the South, of Fire and of Doing, depart now in beauty and in strength. Ruak Itzah Nlame.

All reply:

Blessed be.

Repeat in the West Quarter, with the Priestess saying:

Lords of the West, of Water and of Daring, depart now in beauty and in strength. Ruak Itzah Nlame.

All reply:

Blessed be.

The Priestess draws last dismissing pentagram at the North Quarter and then returns to the South of the altar.

The Priestess puts her ahtame down on the floor and all follow suit.

The Priestess says:

Always remember, all is only to and for and from love.

All reply:

Love is the divine which exists in all of us.

The Priest says:

Blessed be.

All reply:

Blessed be.

All may hug and kiss is so desired.

Guided Meditation to the Old Forest
The Starting Point to the Other Three Meditations

Speaker:
Close your eyes. Get as comfortable as possible. Relax, breathing slowly and deeply, slowly and deeply. Feel as each breath relaxes you further. Each breath in, long and slow. Each breath out, long and slow. Relaxing you.

Focus on your breathing, allowing all your thoughts to drift away, all the concerns of the day. Feel every part of your body beginning to relax, any tensions also melting away.

Relax. Relax. Long slow breaths. Each breath filling you with peace, with a beautiful calm. No concerns, no worries, no fears. Just this moment. Just the sound of my voice.

We are about to journey, leaving this world behind in order to go to another world and to return once more to our own. As has been done in the past, as has been done many times before. Part of you already knows the way. Part of you already knows what to do. For you have done this in the past. You have done this many times before.

See now or imagine that you see that you are in the Old Forest at night. There are trees all around you, great old trees, some of them so big that it would take forty people to hold hands all around their trunk. Trees that are a thousand years old, two thousand. Their branches seemingly stretch to the sky, creating a thick canopy of leaves overhead. Creating a very private and familiar space.

You know these trees. They are oak trees, King Oaks, magickal and powerful. The guardian trees of the forest. Through their leaves you can catch the occasional glimpse of the bright swirl of stars in the night sky. Constellations that tell a story for the stars are familiar, too. Through their branches, you can see the moon, full and bright and mysterious as always. The moon which calls us to our rites.

The leaves of the trees are a dark green, so dark that from a distance they might appear almost black. There is moss growing on the trunks of the trees, moss that is a vivid green even in the dark. Long strands of ivy hang down from some of the tree branches, forming shrouds of green and shadow. Red and ghostly white mushrooms grow among the grass and upon the roots of the trees and up their great trunks.

The air is fresh and cool on your skin. You can smell the rich damp of the earth beneath your feet. The ground is covered with fallen leaves and grass and large white and grey stones rise up out the earth all around you, the visible bones of the Earth Mother. These stones are old, as well, remnants from the last age of ice.

It is still and silent all around you. There are no bird sounds, no animal sounds, even the wind is quiet. As if the forest is holding its breath, as if it is waiting...for something. For this moment, perhaps. For us to be here.

Look around you and see now that you are not alone amongst the great oak trees. See that you have not come here alone this night. Those of the circle are here with you, and they also wait.

Name is here and *name*. (Slowly use this time to name and include all the people in the circle.)

We are all here. We are all waiting. We have come here with purpose and with need, with joy and love in our hearts.

We are Witches. We are *Sorgitza*. We are of the Blood.

This place is ever and always our home upon the earth. It is our foundation and our beginning, our heart song and our dream soul. It is our safe place and our sanctuary and it is from here that we shall journey further.

From here, the circle in the heart of the Old Forest. From the circle of our hearts and of all the spirits we share this world with.

For the Women to Journey to the Underworld

The men should softly hum or chant, perhaps quietly sing a song that has been chosen beforehand—one that either reflects the need or that has become familiar to this particular time and group. This should be done softly enough so that it does not disrupt the rest or so that the speaker cannot be easily heard by those who journey. Eventually, the start of this sound may prove enough to trigger the opening of the mouth of the cave that the women shall enter, but until that point is reached for all concerned, singing or chanting or humming should be done. A quiet drumbeat can also be used, slow and calming.

One chant that may be used for this purpose is:

Root and bone
Root and bone
Down and down
And down we (you) go.

Or

Root and bone
Vine and stone
Down and down
And down we (you) go.

Speaker:

This night we are in need of (healing) (channeling) so the women of the circle shall journey further. They will go from this place into the land of the Underworld. While the men of the circle remain here to guard and to protect, to lend their aid in the return of those who dare travel tonight.

The men will step back to the edge of the grove, where they begin to chant or sing or hum softly. (a cue for the men to begin their song or chanting) The women shall now step together into the middle of the grove, forming a circle together.

In the center of the circle, in the center of the grove of Oaks, a hole slowly begins to spiral open in the ground before you. It widens and deepens as you watch, going down and down, revealing the black and rich heart of the earth. Opening the door through which you shall travel tonight.

As you approach the opening, you can see a ladder going down into the darkness below. A ladder formed of tangled and knotted tree roots and of vines, with rungs made of bone. One by one, you step onto the ladder and begin to slowly and carefully climb downwards.

At first, there is nothing but earth and roots around you, but as you descend this gives way to rock and stone, the bones of *Maman Ehrta*, of Mother Earth. She welcomes you with all the love and familiarity of one who is your truest Mother, who has long known and loved you and your kind.

Down and down you climb. Down and down you go. Deeper and deeper into the embrace of the earth. The tangled roots and vines of the ladder creak gently with each step you make downwards. The damp scent of the earth fills the air around you, a rich and familiar smell.

Your bare feet touch the bones of your ancestors as you climb downwards. They touch those who have come this way before you, who have descended before you.

Down and down you climb, deeper and deeper into the ground. A gentle glow begins to rise up from below, yellow-green, warm and welcoming. You descend towards it, down and down and down, until you finally step off the ladder and into a great cave.

The cave is lit by soft light coming from pale-green and glowing moss beneath your feet. The walls of the cave around you are gleaming, wet with moisture, and they contain swirls of pale stone and reddish mineral. A curtain of glimmering stalactites hangs over your head, their tips dripping crystal water onto the floor below. You can hear the soft sound of running water somewhere in the distance.

In the very center of the cave there is a great stone altar, one carved of living rock. On the center of the altar there sits the skull of an ancient bear. The bone of the skull is yellowed and worn, with great teeth and huge empty eye sockets. The remnants of red clay paint the skull here and there, symbols long worn away by time.

A circle of long bones surrounds the bear skull, each pointing directly at the middle as through the skull stood within the center of a wheel.

You approach the altar and choose one of the long bones. As you lift it up before you, the far end bursts into sudden flame, casting a brilliant white light all around you. A light that reminds you of the heart of the stars.

You can now see a passage leading off from the cave at the far end, a dark mouth which you know you need to enter. One by one, you walk into the passage, holding your bone torch up before you to light the way. The passage is narrow and winding and the floor of glitters beneath your feet.

You turn and spiral with the path, feeling the weight of the earth over your heads, going deeper and deeper. The sound of water grows steadily louder the further that you go, until another cave opens up before you, one even larger than the last.

There are figures painted on the walls in red and white and black paint, most so old that you can only barely make out the outlines of the animals and people they are meant to represent. The cave goes up and up over your heads, up into a darkness that none of the torches can penetrate.

In the center of the cave there lies a pool of black water, so deep, so dark, that no light seems to be able to touch it. The pool is fed by a small spring which is trickling out of the mouth of a carved serpent on the far wall of the cave. The body of the serpent forms a figure eight, the symbol of eternity, and the eyes of the serpent are set with stones the color of blood.

You step up to the edge of the pool and look down at the surface of it. No water you have ever seen has ever looked so still or so black as this. It feels as though there may be no bottom to the pool, no end. But even as you stare at the water, the surface ripples for a moment, as though something moved in it just below the surface.

You kneel down by the edge of the pool, close enough to touch the water. There is something in the water, you know it. It's what you came here for tonight, why you journeyed to this place.

You have come for what is needed, a way of healing or a message. It can take many shapes…the form of a word, a symbol, a ritual, an herb, a chant, a spell, a prayer. One of them will show the way. One of them will tell you what you need to know.

It is time. Reach into the dark waters. Touch the blood of the Earth. And remember…

(At this point, the Speaker should remain silent for a length of time.)

It is time to leave the pool now, time to return to the world above with what you have received, with what you have learned.

One by one, you stand and lift up your torches again. You turn away from the dark pool and enter the winding passageway once more.

Back and back, down the narrow path you return, traveling once more through the depths of earth and stone. Back and back, you walk, the light proceeding ahead of you, shrinking down to blackness behind you.

Until finally, you are once more back in the cave where the altar sits, where the ancient bear skull awaits your return. As you approach the altar, the bone torch in your hand flickers and dims and goes out. You replace it on the altar in the same position you took it from before, once more making a wheel around the bear skull. It has served its purpose this night.

The yellow-green glow from the moss guides you back to the vine and bone ladder and, one by one, you take hold of it once more. You begin to climb up, one step at a time. Up and up, the ladder creaking softly as you go.

Up and up, past stone and past earth and roots. Climbing back to the world above. Climbing out of the tender embrace of the Mother. Up and up you go, until at last you can see the faint gleam of moonlight above you. Until you can smell the fresh night air above and hear the sounds of the men as they welcome you back, as they guide you home again.

And you are feeling lighter and lighter as well, so light that you feel you could all but fly up the last few rungs of the ladder.

The night and the moon and the forest welcomes you as you emerge from the earth, as you stand on the grass in the center of the grove once more. The men end their chanting and come to stand with you, glad at your safe return.

For a long moment, you all stand there, men and women together, a circle between the earth and the sky. Between the world above and the world below. The white moon high overhead and the stars glimmering between the branches of the trees, revealing patterns that have of old traced themselves into your rituals, into your hearts.

FoR The Men to JouRney into the OveRwoRld

Speaker:

This night we are in need of works of magick so the men of the circle shall journey further. They will go from this place into the land of the Overworld, the world above. While the women of the circle remain here to guard and to protect, to lend their aid in the return of those who dare travel tonight.

The women will step back to the edge of the grove, where they begin to chant or sing or hum softly. (a cue for the women to begin their song or chanting) The men step together into the middle of the grove, forming a circle together.

One chant that may be used for this purpose is:

Fire and light
Flame and air
Up and up
We (you) go, we (you) dare.

Or

Up and up and up we (you) go
Into the sky
From the world below
To climb the hill of heaven's bright
To seek the heights
To know the light.

In the center of the grove a large granite stone slowly begins to rise up from out of the ground. It is ancient and pitted and cragged, carved by the passage of time and the elements of wind and water. Ancient symbols, some of them so faded they are nearly invisible, are also carved onto its great sides.

The stone seems almost to hum with a life of its own and, one by one, you are drawn towards it. Each of you reach out to the stone, finding it rough and smooth at the same time, both hot and cold to the touch. There are cracks in the stone, cracks big enough to slip your hands and feet into, and you use them as you begin to climb.

The top of the stone is very wide, wide enough that all of you can once more stand together in a circle. As you stand there, your eyes are drawn upwards to the sky. The stars shimmer above, forming familiar patterns in the darkness. As you stare at them, they begin to swirl and flash across the heavens, forming a web of light, an electric storm. You begin to feel light and lighter, as though you could go flying up into the sky at any moment.

A ladder suddenly drops down into the center of your circle. The ladder glimmers and shines like the stars, almost as though it were made of light itself. Its strands are braided from gold and silver and its rungs fashioned out of some dark metal that seems to glow softly from within.

One after the other, you begin to climb the ladder. One by one, you begin to go up into the sky, the world above.

Up and up you climb, leaving the rock and the grove below. The Earth gently recedes beneath your feet as you ascend and the ladder thrums softly as you climb. Up and up, higher and higher, the open air cool and fresh around you. And you feel lighter and lighter as you go, as though you were becoming one with the air and the sky.

Mist begins to gather around you, fine and cool and damp. White and silver, a thin trail of clouds sweeps across the moon, obscuring the stars behind them. Higher and higher now, the air thin, but still breathable, and now you are among the clouds. They're wet on your skin, tasting of rain not yet fallen to the Earth.

And then the clouds and mist part at last to reveal the land above, the Overworld. They part to reveal the crystal hills of the heavens, the mountains of the sky.

The ladder ends and you step off into this new world, feeling it softly yielding beneath your feet, yet firm enough to hold you up. The sky seems impossibly close over your head, its darkness fixed with glittering gems of all sizes and colors. Stars, galaxies, planets, some familiar and some strange.

In the distance, towards the crystal mountains, a blue-white light shimmers and flickers and you are drawn towards it. You walk towards it through an ever changing, ever shifting, landscape of things seen and half-seen. A maze of mist and shadow, one where nothing is quite what it seems.

At last, the mountains lie directly before you. There is a great stone stairway leading into their heart, curving into their depths. You begin to walk up the steps and they are wide and deep, as though giants once walked here. Giants and heroes of legend and Gods of days long past.

The stairs takes you to a temple set within a deep valley, one surrounded on all sides steep cliff-faces, by the very bones of the mountain. The temple is open to the sky and ringed by eight tall columns, four of them red and four white. A hot blue flame rises up from the top of each column, giving off the terrible, sweet smell of sulphur.

In the center of the ring of columns, there is an altar fashioned of gold and white stone. On the altar, floating just above its surface, you see a large brightly glowing orb of light.

You are drawn to the light. As you look into it colors and shapes and figures appear and disappear, shades and shadows of what is, what may be, what once was. It is at the same time a mirror and a light and a flame and a polished shield. It is fire and ice and light and shadow.

You circle the altar, you circle the flame, feeling both its intense heat and its terrible chill. You know that what you desire is within the fire. That within the center of the flames you will find what you came here for tonight, why you journeyed to this place.

You know the knowledge with burn you, but you have come for what is needed. A work of magick which can take many shapes...the form of a word, a symbol, a ritual, a chant, a spell, a prayer. One of them will show the way. One of them will tell you what you need to know.

It is time. Reach out to touch the flame, to grasp the fire of the heavens. And remember...

(At this point, the Speaker should remain silent for a length of time.)

It is time to let go of the fire now, time to return to the world below with what you have received, with what you have learned. Step away from the flames and walk out of the circle of columns, back onto the wide stairs that led you here.

Back and back you go, down the stairway through the mountains. Back and back, across the plains of mist and cloud, shifting and ever changeable. The crystal mountains of the heavens shrinking behind you, until they disappear at last into the mist and darkness behind you.

Until finally, you see the top of the gold and silver ladder and, one, by one, you take hold of it once more. You begin to climb down, one step at a time. Down and down, through damp and cool darkness, until the clouds give way to the open air, revealing the moon once more. Until you can see the Earth spread out beneath you like a distant pattern of light and shadow, a compass map.

Down and down, climbing back to the world you have known, the world where you were born. Down and down, feeling heavier and heavier now as you descend. The forest rising up to meet you now, the top of the great stone.

One by one, you step off the ladder and back onto the stone. It hums gently beneath your feet, even as you smell the earth around you and hear the sounds of the women as they welcome you back, as they guide you home again.

The gold and silver ladder, the ladder of the heavens, disappears back into the sky and you climb down the side of the stone, seeing now that its patterns are similar to those etched into the night sky. The stone once more sinks into the ground, leaving no mark behind.

The night and the moon and the forest welcomes you as you stand on the grass in the center of the grove once more, back where you began. The women end their chanting and come to stand with you, glad at your safe return.

For a long moment, you all stand there, men and women together, a circle between the earth and the sky. Between the world above and the world below. The white moon high overhead and the stars glimmering between the branches of the trees, revealing patterns that have of old traced themselves into your rituals, into your hearts.

FoR All to JouRney to Benevento

A chant that may be used:

Io itzahtzak
Away away
To play the game
We will go
We must fly
Open the door
Show the way.

Or:

Io itzahtzak
Away away
Gebhest we call
Gebhest we name
Open the door
Show the way.

Speaker:

Together we step into the center of the grove, here in the heart of the Old Forest. Together, we form a circle and ready ourselves to journey further, to go the Witches' place, to Benevento, to play the Game.

(All but the Speaker may begin chanting softly at this point, either one of the chants above or some other chosen for that purpose.)

To the North-East of our circle a door opens into the very fabric of reality, bright light shining into our midst. A light so white that it is dark at the core. A tall male shape appears within the doorway, a figure dressed all in black. He is the guide and the opener of the way. We know His name as we know His purpose here, what we ask of Him this night.

All around you the air begins to shimmer now, colors flashing and shivering across your skin. Colors we have seen before and colors we have never known before. A heat begins to grow inside your chest and your flesh suddenly feels too small, too tight. You feel a desperate need to move, to do, to go…while, at the same time, you desire to sleep. You can barely keep your eyes open.

Suddenly, the light and heat flashes all around you and now your totem stands before you. It may be an animal, a bird, a plant, whatever it is that calls to you and has been long a part of you and of your blood. It is here now to bear you away, to take you to the Game, to the place of Benevento, to the Witches' Sabbat of old.

You climb on your totem and it bears you up. The Guide beckons from the open door and you feel His touch upon you. You enter the door.

The Void lies all around you, eternity above and below, and you move through it on the back of your power, your dream. Light and darkness rush past, colors stream by, worlds and universes seen and unseen, strange and familiar. And yet there is no light, no darkness, no color at all, nothing to touch and nothing to hold onto.

But then you begin to smell the distant scent of flowers and know that you are close. A mist rises up around you and suddenly there solid ground beneath you once more. Your totem, your power, has brought you where you needed to go.

The mist begins to lift, pulling back to reveal a wide meadow or field. The meadow is filled from one end to the other with roses. Pale pink roses with only five petals each, a golden light, glowing softly at the heart of each flower. Their soft, sweet scent rises up around you, making you feel warm and welcome. You know this place. You have always known this place.

In the distance, you see a castle or a great house. While, nearer to hand, a tall tree stands, its branches reaching all the way up into the silvery sky. A spring lies beneath it, fresh water rushing and bubbling up from beneath the roots of the tree. The water looks cool and clear, healing water. Water from the depths of time. Water from the cave of the beginnings.

It is time. This is where you play the Game. The Game which is not a Game.

Across the field from you, you now see there is a whole line of other Witches, men and women together, each of them riding upon their own totem. Eagles and cats and wrens and snakes and wolves. Stags and salmon and spiders and bolts of lightning torn down from the sky. BEasts and birds and fish and symbols of every kind and sort that could possibly be imagined.

They are here to play the Game, as well. They are here to battle and to fEast, and to alter worlds. They are here as you are here, to be with your own kin, with your own family. Those of your own time and place, and those scattered across all of history.

Witches all, you have gathered here. Witches all, both the living and the dead, this is your place. This is your home. This is where you come from and this is where you will always return to. Your power lies here, your power and your destiny.

It is time. The Game awaits you. Your family awaits you. You enter the field...

(At this point, the Speaker should remain silent for a length of time.)

It's time to end the Game now, time to return to the world where you came from. To your own time and place. The mist begins to gather upon the field again, obscuring the great house, obscuring the tree and the spring below. The smell of roses begins to grow faint and distant, though you know their scent will never quite leave you and that you will always remember it.

The Void opens up before you again, dark and distant, cold and empty, but you seek your way home with confidence and surety. You seek your own time, your own place, your own world. The Earth of your Blood, of your ancestors and of those yet to come. Stars and planets fly past you, times known and unknown, selves you never were and selves you might have been.

Through them all, you seek your own self, the place where you belong. The darkness parts, revealing a distant and familiar light, and you rush towards it, eager to be home again. You pass back through the gate, back to your own world, your own time, to where and when you are meant to be.

As the night welcomes you back and the moon and the great trees of the Old Forest. As your brothers and sisters welcome you home.

For a long moment, you all stand there, men and women together, a circle between the earth and the sky. Between the world above and the world below. The white moon high overhead and the stars glimmering between the branches of the trees, revealing patterns that have of old traced themselves into your rituals, into your hearts.

Conclusion to the Guided Meditations ~ Return From the Old Forest

(The Speaker judges when it is time to return, then begins the following piece.)

You are children of the night sky and of the earth. Both have fixed themselves deep within you, never to be lost. You are at peace here. You remember this place. It will never leave you, no matter how far you wander. It will always be your home, your peace, your sanctuary, a part of your body, blood, heart, and spirit.

Do not fear, do not forget, but remember.

(The Speaker should allow for a few moments of silence here.)

But is time to leave now, time to return. Though the peace of this place shall remain with you, as all here shall remain with you. An unbreakable bond. An eternal circle. Part of the cycle of life and time, of love and eternity.

Listen to the sound of my voice now as I count backwards from ten to one. As I count, you will begin to wake and to stir, to return to yourselves. To leave the Old Forest and the circle within.

Ten. Back and back, we shall return.

Nine. Each of us beginning to stir, to wake.

Eight. Peaceful and knowing and strong, we will come here again.

Seven. Rested and hopeful for what is to begin.

Six. Becoming more and more awake now.

Five. Returning to the circle that we all share.

Four. Remembering what the journey has shown us.

Three. More and more aware, ready to face the future together.

Two. Our eyes slowly coming open, able to see.

One. And we are here and back and awake and aware and with each other.

All should wake and stretch at this point, getting back into awareness of their bodies and of the world around them. At this point, if you have the time, you should all share your experiences and write down as much as you can remember, especially any messages, symbols, or information that you have received. You can either take the time to do this while you are still in ritual, or do it immediately after you close your circle. People should also be encouraged to write down their experiences in their own personal journals if they keep any.

To Dance the Blood

Do not despair, but dance!
Do not weep, but dance!
Do not tremble with fear, but dance!
Do not forget—dance!
It is the first promise and the first lesson in one.
From the beginning of time and unto the end, which are, after all, the same—to be a
Witch is to dance.
And remember your shadow dances with you.

Dark moon, dark tides, and part of me asks what stirs this night, what stirs within our blood…even as part of me already knows and welcomes what's to come. The wine tasted of blood, which is as it should be, as it used to be. It tasted of the blood of the Gods and the Blood of the Witches and we drank deep and then danced.

We spun round and round, feeling the wine imparting life as much as it also had about it the bittersweet flavor of death. But then we all knew that each is a bud upon the same tree, one opening only to have another close. That time spins like a top, from life to death and from death to life. As we, we the Witches, those of the Blood, exist on both sides, as Witches in life and as Other in death.

So we ran and so we drank and so we danced and so we spun…a flowering bloom. Each of us bare of foot in order to best feel the Earth, our Mother, as we danced the round of old. Flesh pressing to the Earth, each step was a connection to the ground and to the past. As each leap was a flight into the wild unknown, into the future. Leap and dance, round and about, the dances of Witches by nature reflect nature; they are always about the powers of life and death and of rebirth.

Some sorts of dances have to them the quality of the God, dances that mimic journeys made to strange and terrible lands in order to bring back wonders. Just as there are Goddess dances, dances that are rounds of rising desire and the bounty of the earth and the sea. Finally, there are dances that reflect the joining of men and of women, of the Gods and of Witches, of the heavens and of the earth, of the light and of the dark, of spirit and flesh. A joining that is both a beginning and an ending.

But there is yet another sort of dance that Witches do, one that they must do. There is the dancing to remember. For to be a Witch is to dance, and when a Witch dances, or one who has it within them to be a Witch, then they recall who and what they are. When a Witch dances he or she becomes a flame, part of the eternal fire. Every time they dance, the Blood is called to remember what it is. For the dance stirs the Blood. It awakens it and this awakening spreads both to the future and to memories long past. While the dance itself lies at the core of the ripple, a stone flung into still water—and so a Witch lives to dance and dances to live.

The dance bestows a certain lightness of heart as much as it stirs the fire that sleeps within the Blood. This bright flame, this lightness of spirit, electrifies the body and thrills the soul. Miracles and magicks spin out from it in all directions, for once linked to faith and to knowledge, anything is possible. You walk in the world, but you dance in the dream, and an awakened Witch embodies both at the same time, bringing the two together as one. They become the doorway, standing with one foot in one land and one foot in the other. For this, a Witch is forged; it is both their greatest duty and their greatest pleasure.

You may have the remnants of the old Witch Blood in your veins, but in order to be *of the Blood*, in order to find your way to the *first circle*, it is required that the Blood be awakened within your body. It must be stirred up, excited, and turned to sacred fire in your veins, until the spirit itself becomes as intoxicated. To know who and what you are in your deepest heart of hearts, you must dance. If you are to be a Witch you *have* to dance. There is no way around it. This is the most important step of all in the recovery of what was and what needs to be again. To dance and so to wake and so to remember…

This is the true secret of resurrection as those who sleep the sleep of death do not wholly return, even though they have been born back to the flesh, unless they are also born again to the fire. The fire which is part of a Witch's true nature and power. Being that Witches are of the South Quarter, Fire and Doing find expression through their blood and through the actions of the Witch.

This fire can rise up and restore all the powers once thought lost, even those powers denied by many today as ever having existed except in the minds of those too primitive to understand the ways of reason and science. The fire of the Blood is the fire of the mind and the fire of the heart...the doorway to the Second Sight which is needed in order to perform much of the ancient magicks.

To dance the dance of the Blood, the dance of remembrance, the dance that stirs and shakes you to wakefulness, is to become a Witch in body, mind, and spirit. It is a lightening of the body, an expansion of the mind, a bubbling up of love and light and laughter in the spirit. It rises up until it becomes too great to contain and the consciousness, the spirit, must fling itself free of the heavy weight of flesh.

You dance around the core of who you are, seeing all of your self, past, present, and future, and seeing also your vital place in the great web of the universe. You dance until the flesh sleeps and the spirit awakes to its nature and floats free of your body, a bright spark, a firefly, Witch fire, withy glow, light and ethereal as thistledown. Only then, may you and those with you pass through the door to the worlds unseen, to Benevento, to the Game, to the field, to the Witches sacred World Mountain. Where the Gods and Witches everywhere and everywhen await you.

The dance is, of old, the way for the *Sorgitza* to remember the Blood and the ways of the Blood. It *is* an intoxication of the spirit and so much more than that. If you Dance the Blood for a full year and a day, who knows what might result? It is the first step along the road to Benevento, to the Witches Sabbat place. To where the Game is played, the game which is not a game.

Ritual for Dancing the Blood

Each person should drink deeply of the cup of red wine, either their own cup or a shared coven cup. Afterwards, all dance in a circle, fast or slow, sharing a measured pace with their hands held or dancing wildly. Or you may choose to start off slow and build to a faster pace. This can be done in silence or, if you are in a place where it is safe to make a lot of noise, you can cry out as you desire or are moved to. Songs or chants may also be used, though it is a good idea to continue to use the same one so that it will become familiar to you and not distract you from the dance. The simpler the song or the chant the more powerful it can prove. Rhyming ones are best of all.

The following may be used:

Sorgae sorgitzak arahnak orono
Sorgae sorgitzak arahnak oray

All this being said, it will take at least and year and day to succeed fully in learning to Dance the Blood. But the more often you dance, the more success you will meet, though if not done passionately and often it will most certainly take even longer than a year and a day. For, in the Old Days, there was more in the cup than simple wine.

Orono ze zoma
Orono ze arahnak
Itzah arahnak
Itzah sorgitzak
Itzah oray

To Ride to the Sabbat

The bright serpent coiled about the great tree
His heart's blood whispers secrets to thee
Of corn and of glade beneath the warm sun
Love given and found for what is begun
Lit from the candle held high in his crown
Blue fire calls to senses unbound
To hie to the pounding of drums in the night
Where he of the land shall again lead the rite.

We ran from the hill as if madness were behind us, as if we were chasing desire. We ran to the Sabbat...as was done in years long ago. My heart was loud, my pulse wicked and fast. I could smell the oil I had anointed myself with; even through my clothes, it was fire. Where it touched my skin it created a burning impulse to run and leap and laugh, to be a part of this moment, of the chase, to be wild and free at last.

I grinned, unable to stop myself. I raced, chasing others, chasing something as yet unseen. My blood felt alive, more alive than it had ever felt before. The past, the future, none of that mattered—only the now, only the chase, and I ran as though I was the hunter and hunted both. I knew the God's power as my own, the wanton sensation of blood and wine, the dappled skin of a faun, of the mingling of wild-haired women and the lords of the forest. I ran and ran with the voice of the God in my mind, his drums my heart, his blood my vine.

The race seemed to last forever, and yet it took no time at all. I could have kissed every one I ran with; I wanted to touch them, to know them intimately...and, the strangest thing was that I felt this odd desire to consume what I loved. I felt as though I could have just eaten them I wanted them so very much. It would have been the highest high of love— to consume what you desired the most, to make it a part of yourself. They laughed as they ran, too, and looked back at me with eyes of fire. As if they all wanted to be eaten, as if they wanted me in the same feral and ferocious way. As though we were both predator and prey at the same time.

But then, unsurprisingly, the Lord of the Hunt ran with us. He ran within us. We had stepped from our world to His when we stood in a circle on the hill in order to receive his fire, the fire that now surged in our veins and urged us to run, run, run. It was a gift once stolen from the Gods, from the heavens, and now it was ours again, at least for a little while. The gift of sublime life.

Others ran with us, Witches of the past and of the future, joining us from the land of ghosts and shadows. But then each hunt is the same hunt, as every chase is eternal. The God lends His madness and his life...and we are made immortal for it. Who can ask for more than that? Who can ask for more than one bright shining moment of being truly alive? And when are you more alive than when you stand upon the brink of death?

This can be done before each Sabbat, and not only does it raise a lot of energy, but it gets you into the right ritual mood. If possible, it's a good idea to begin upon a hill a little ways from where you intend to raise your circle. Running through the woods at night can also be exhilarating and mood altering if you have the place to do so. Of course, it's not strictly necessary to run, but if you walk instead, you should all walk with purpose and resolve, letting the night and the scent of the oil and the company you keep seep into your mind and body, into your blood. Singing or chanting as you walk also lends to the atmosphere, but you can also choose to yell or scream if it's safe to do so.

Ritual For Riding to the Sabbat

Everyone but the Priestess gathers upon the top of a hill or in the woods and anoints their body with some form of perfumed oil. You may use whatever oil seems to stir your senses best and you can share the same one between you or use one that is personal to you alone. It should be put on the pulse points such as the back of the knees, the bend of the elbow, behind the ear, or you may rub it all over your body or even over your clothing. If you are using an oil that can burn the naked skin, such as oils with cinnamon in it, then be careful where you apply it and use it sparingly.

These words may be said as people are putting on the oil, or shortly thereafter, by either the Priest or a chosen speaker:

You are a star fallen to earth, yet you remain one with the heavens. Your nature is fire—from fire you come and to fire you shall return. The breath of the wind is your brother (sister), with water and the salt of the earth to purify all that you do. You are a Priest (Priestess) of the world, brought down to heal and guide and protect all those who have not yet tasted the dew of heaven.

Do not forget. Dance and sing and make merry, for these are your best and brightest gifts. Drink deep of joy as much as of sorrow, and know how there is never one without the other for one mirrors the other.

There is nothing else. There is only this—love beyond imagining, love beyond measuring, love eternal and everlasting. To live in love is to be alive and to never die. To live in love is be a Shining One. To recall your days among the stars.

Do not fail to dance. Do not fear to sing. Make merry in all that you say and do and your heart shall be lightened so that you will become as thistledown blown upon the wind. Run and laugh and cry until your heart bursts into blossoms, into light, into the dawn. Into tomorrow and yesterday.

Be who you are and all shall be made known to you and it shall become as you, for you are a child of the Gods and the starry heavens and there is no greater promise than that.

No greater joy. No greater hope.

Now, run, run, run…

The Priest breaks the circle with a shout or a clap of his hands, or by simply yelling "go" or "now," and everyone runs for the place where the circle is going to be cast. The Priest should come last, inspiring the runners to greater speed. If agreed to beforehand, he may even lightly strike people with a leafy branch, though playfully, of course. This is the source of the old term "and the devil take the hindmost."

If you've all decided beforehand that it will be more of a walk than a run, someone can be chosen to lead the procession—possibly carrying a lit torch or even a stang—but the Priest should always come last. As the Priestess remains to greet them, the Priest should always be the last to arrive. The Priestess is the only one who does not take part in the run to the Sabbat, for she is the one who waits for them to enter into the place where the circle will be created.

You can also use candles or torches to light your way, though there should be a bucket of water or sand placed near the end of the run or procession so that they can safely be put out. Masks may be worn and people can ride brooms or staffs according to their desire. It will, of course, depend on whether or not you all intend to run, in which case torches or brooms might get in the way. Also, the location might dictate whether or not you can have torches, especially if it is in a park of some kind and not private property.

The important part is not so much the wearing of masks or the waving of torches, but using the run or the procession as a pre-curser to ritual.

Connecting to the land

Where the bone God goes, fire goes too...
Lost in the mists of time before time, there existed the bone God and the bone
Goddess, She of the caves, She who was ancient even before the rise of the Earth
Mother.
Together, they walked among those who were not yet human, for whom the gift of fire
would make human.
While those of the air came to earth also as fire, as living flame, and with them came
the first gifts—for Pandora was not so much a maiden as a promise. And Hope, her
brightest star of all, the dawn of heaven, the flame in the heart, the song of praise
raised to the beauty of the flesh that spirit chose to cloak itself in.
Breath and fire, blood and bone...so all things came to be, whether they truly know
themselves or not.
And so remembering is the key, and the hardest promise of all to keep.
Even though it is always near, as they are always near, deep, deep inside us, where we
are yet kin with the oldest ones of all—the lord of skull and crossed bones and the
lady of the caves.

A Legend of the Sorgitza

Dirt is more than just dirt. It is more than just what we walk on or what we grow things in. The earth of a place retains the essence of a place. It is imbued with a piece of the spirit of a place. The spirits of trees, rocks, earth, flowers and all growing things are tied to where they reside. They carry the imprint of the land inside them, and are connected to the spirit of the land—a conscious and living spirit which has a life and purpose of its own. Of course, Earth spirits being of a different nature than our own, they do not exactly think or react the same way as we do, which can make them hard to relate to or understand.

For one thing, they take a much longer view of the world. Time, for them, is not measured at the frantic pace that most of us are used to. This long-term viewpoint also lends itself to having somewhat different goals and ways of going about accomplishing those goals. Seeing the big picture comes natural to them because they think less in terms of months or years, than in centuries and eons. Small wonder, they don't always sweat the small stuff.

The thing is that the small stuff may sometimes include things humans consider important or valuable so that trying to make spirits of the Earth understand just why you want this or that to happen can prove to be a trying challenge and one that you may not always succeed at. But there are benefits to this. The spirits of some places are old, so very old that we truly cannot comprehend what exactly that means and with that great age comes great patience, far more patience than most of us could ever hope for. Though even that great patience is not inexhaustible.

The greatest Earth spirit of all—so great an Earth spirit that She is a Goddess—is Mother Earth Herself and She is very patient. In fact, She loves us and nurtures us, as She loves all that live here, for they and we are all flesh of Her flesh, bone of Her bone. But as She loved the dinosaurs once upon a time, that does not mean that any of Her children are invulnerable or that we today are immune to the eventual consequences of what is being done in the name of greed, ignorance, or progress. When we hurt the Earth, we hurt our Mother, and even a mother will only put up with just so much pain and disrespect.

It is high time for the Western world to reclaim responsibility and to learn to think long term, to see the future as being created today. A future that needs to be there, not just for the Earth, but for all the children of the Earth. Some native traditions think seven generations ahead, and where could they have learned such long term vision but from the very land itself? But then if we are not truly tied to the land, if we cannot hear the voice of the Earth, how can we understand how to live in proper accord with it.

People used to be accustomed to being bound to the land they lived on and it was a natural and normal state for them. They knew their lives relied upon it—particularly upon its continued fertility—and that the relationship was one of mutual need, of mutual give and take. Now, however, most people have cut these ties and have wandered far from their original homes, far from the wellsprings of power which once renewed their bodies. And most do not know how, or even that they *should* connect to the place where they reside now. In fact, in some cases, they have wandered so very far that they are, in some essence, lost...even to themselves.

They no longer know the way back and they don't know how to go forward, how to reconnect to the Earth which lives and breathes beneath their feet. Her heartbeat is a dim and distant memory, one that is hard to hear unless you learn the secrets of silence. But we need Mother Earth. Our very flesh is made of Her and the same way in which we walk upon Her body, She walks with us wherever we go, whatever we do. She is with us when our buildings reach upwards to the sky. In this way, She reaches to the sky. When mankind walked upon the moon for the very first time, She touched the moon with them.

She is always a part of us, but this relationship needs to be acknowledged and renewed, as all good relationships must from time to time. We should not take Her for granted, nor our place in Her favors, or in the favors of the other spirits of the land. Instead, we need to form a link to the place where we reside, to learn to hear the voice of the spirits who imbue it with life. We need to create and keep a living and viable relationship, both for ourselves and for future generations. We have to begin to ask and to listen to those voices once more.

One of the reasons why it is harder to do magick today is because the level of vibration is too heavy, and this heaviness stems from humans lack of belief that such things are possible, even natural to our existence. One must fight that weight of disbelief, both what is ingrained in the world and what is ingrained in our own minds from the conscious and unconscious expectations of society. In some places, however, places where the power nodes and wellsprings lie, the vibration levels are higher and so magick still comes easier. It floats and flows and sings through the land, as it would seek to float and flow and sing through your veins if you but let it.

The power of the land sleeps inside us, but sometimes places sleep and they need to be awakened as much as people. Many Earth spirits have awakened already and some have never slept at all. But of those that sleep still, when they wake up they will seek to understand this time and the people who now live here, and some may be less than pleased at what has gone on while they slept. Some will be confused because they do not understand how any people can live apart from the Earth and not be respectful towards it.

In part, it's because we've lost the innate knowledge of our ancestors, who understood the importance of creating and maintaining a living link to the land, especially since this relationship was necessary for their very survival. Modern science has "taught" us that such a link is not necessary, choosing instead to treat the Earth as though it were just some sort of machine, much like modern medicine tends to treat the human body. This is a short sighted and simplistic viewpoint and one that has, in part, led to disease both in humans and in the Earth Herself. It has led to a decided lack of balance.

To reconnect, we need to contact and connect with the spirits of the Earth, as well as with the natural wellsprings of power that lie in the land where we live. Rivers form either boundaries or wellsprings, depending upon whether they are "male" or "female" in nature. Male rivers such as "Old Man River," the Mississippi, form boundaries between one area of the earth and another, areas which are fed by the energy of the attendant wellspring. So the wellspring of the Eastern United States lies East of the Mississippi and the wellspring of the Western part of the country lies West of the Mississippi in the Black Hills, the sacred lands of the Lakota people.

Back in Europe, however, the Danube or Duna river is female in nature and hence a wellspring and not a boundary. It's the source of power and energy in all the lands that it flows through and once upon a time, the people in those lands knew of Ardwena, the Goddess who claimed it as Her own. Even though the Duna is a river and so of the element of Water, Ardwena is an Earth Goddess. She is also the Goddess who can show us how to rebuild our bond with the Earth and Her spirits, Her energies.

Of course, the Earth spirits themselves have a say in what sort of bond we form with them. Like any relationship, it involves trust building and give-and-take, as well as learning about each other. Earth spirits differ from region to region and so the form of the interaction may also differ from region to region depending upon the shape of their "personalities."

Of the Earth spirits who are awake, some are unhappy over the current state of affairs and may have to be reassured of your good intent. While others just naturally more contrary or difficult to deal with, often reflecting the nature of the land itself. Honesty and humility are watchwords when dealing with the spirits of the Earth. It also pays to learn how to be silent yourself, so that you stand a better chance of hearing them. They can and will give messages, but those messages often come in the form of feelings or symbols, so you have to pay attention. And trust in both them and in your own instincts.

If you want to create a lasting link to the land, then you must put a part of yourself into it. If the bones of your ancestors do not already lie there, if their blood has not flowed into the Earth with the intent of making them and their kin part of the land they live upon, then you are unlikely to already have a connection to it. For it is in this way that families who have lived in a certain area for hundreds of years have made a link with it and with the spirits of the land who dwell there. Their family has become one with the Earth of their ancestors.

In order to form an accord, you need to give some of your blood to the Earth. But you should not do so lightly, knowing that you will be moving away in a year or five years, traveling to live in some other part of the country that is under the auspices of another land spirit. If you do, you will have to change allegiance to the governing spirit of that region, and if you treat such changes lightly—as most of us do today, moving easily from place to place, sometimes across continents—then how can you expect the spirits of the land to take you seriously? How can you expect them to desire to make an alliance with you if you and your family are going to be leaving in what is, to them, a blink of an eye.

Worse still, most people already treat the land these days in a disrespectful way, demanding much and giving little in return, using it up and poisoning it recklessly, heedless and unthinking of the world they shall leave to their own children and to their children's children. It is very selfish not to take several generations into consideration when it comes to dealing with the land and the bounty of the land.

Mother Earth needs to be respected, as do any accords made with Her spirits. Most especially any accord which binds your blood to it and which uses the power of your blood to wake those spirits and to call yourself to their attention.

Ritual for Connecting to the Spirits of the Land

To make this accord, the words matter far less than the action and your intent. But at least three drops of blood should be given to the land, with the feeling and desire of forging a link between yourself and the spirits of the Earth.

For a woman, her moon blood will do—and should be given, at least in some small part every month thereafter to strengthen the bond. But a gift of food or drink can also be offered, or some other gift which you have made yourself. The more personal the gift the better, as it will have stronger ties to you. Though, of course, it is best to give something which shall eventually be dissolved into the land and not harm it.

Bury your offering in the ground or hang it in a tree with raffia or some other sort of twine or cord which is all-natural. Close your eyes and open yourself up to the land that you stand on, to the spirits of the earth. It's not strictly necessary to say anything, simply to hold honest intent in your heart, but if you desire to say a few words, then the following can be used:

This I give
That we shall come to know each other
This I give
That we shall gain an accord
Between fire and earth
This I give
To wake to know to be as one
With the spirits of the earth
Of this place
Ertahlia ensiehta
Ertahlia hostarak
Ensiehta ze zoma
Arahnak ertahlia
Arahnak

If you decide to forge this link to the land, however, you be aware that the land may ask for gifts in the future—as well as give you gifts, which should be accepted with the honor they are due—and that when you travel you may be leaving the territory of the spirit with which you have made an accord, so that you might need to ask permission to enter the land where another spirit presides. It's not as if the spirit would deny you entry, necessarily, but it is simply the proper thing to do and shows that you are both aware of and respectful of the Earth and Her guardian spirits.

There may be a sign after you perform this rite, one that shows you that your offering has been accepted. The land most often contacts us in signs and omens; if we are patient and pay attention to the world around us we can come to "read" their messages. For example, when a link to a local land spirit was formed a few years back, a bald eagle appeared in the skies right overhead and circled three times. At another time, there was the sound of distant drums in the middle of the night. A sound that several of us heard, though we were never quite sure was with our minds or with our ears, even though we all heard the same exact beat.

One way of keeping this contact after it is made is by being sure to touch the land as often as possible, even if you have to dig through snow or ice in the wintertime to do so or by bringing back some of it with you in a jar to your home. Physical contact is very important when you are dealing with the spirits and powers of the Earth.

Beyond the Earth

Soundings of the deep
It rises from the hidden places
Though you can never see its face
You know it is there
You always knew it was there
For it rises inside you as well
Something greater than your skin
Something as large as your soul
We are all more than what we seem
A particle of clear bright sand
Caught between the two angles of the hourglass
All that pours down into a tiny mote
Adrift upon an immortal sea
Footsteps run down the shore
To tease the tides that desire them
But what cannot be washed away is all that remains
Like the relentless bleached bones
Of some monster bEast
Who once consumed a heart
Of molten gold and broken copper
All the pieces that lay scattered
Along the prism of the spine
Of the world.

But what of the Gods who represent powers and principalities that go far beyond the boundaries of this planet? For there are spiritual consciousnesses that are larger and even less understandable at a human level than Mother Earth. We cannot hope to grasp Her in Her entirety—for She is the consciousness of the whole Earth, which includes millions years of history, a history in which we have existed but for the briefest of moments—yet even the Earth is small when compared in turn to the vast expanse of the universe. Even more so if you take into account what lies beyond the purely visible universe, for the Unseen world is greater still.

The expanse of the spiritual universe is immense beyond reckoning, layers upon layers. Generally, we can only handle the smallest glimpse of these realms, being that our physical bodies are limited. Can you pour the whole of the ocean into one tiny speck of sand? Let alone all of space and time into one tiny blue-white planet or into one person standing upon the shores of that planet…yes, you can. But if it lasts more than but a few moments, that speck of sand risks being destroyed, or transformed forever, as sand is forged and fused into glass. Our physical bodies are just not meant to bear such tremendous powers for very long.

When you open that door, so much comes rushing through it that you can only stand so much. Especially as it comes over you in equal parts of ecstasy and fear, joy and pain, a pain that can even take on a physical component. Your heart pounds, your whole body aches, and you don't know whether you feel more like laughing or crying and can even end up doing both at the same time.

But then you want to weep, you want to laugh, you want to shout out to anyone who can hear you—its here, its now, its all around us, can't you see? You shake and shudder and feel so very much that, even as you might want to hold onto it forever—this sensation of the ultimate, this glorious and wonderful moment of understanding—yet you cannot bear to keep it at the same time. You don't want to leave behind that perfect clarity, but yet it hurts too much to stay there. Despite this, it leaves you with the desire to feel it again, to once more walk through that door of perception.

They are ancient gates—joy and terror, pain and pleasure—gates which are meant not just to show you what lies beyond this world, but gates which are reflections of each other. For true beauty is terrible, as God was once said to be terrible or awful. Not because God, or the Divine Source, is a terrible or awful thing in the negative sense of the word, but because you feel awe in the presence of the Divine, sublime awe and sublime terror.

Except that what is "ordinary" and "everyday" is not really, because it's all in our perspective. The world does not really change when the gate opens—you do. You learn to see behind the mask, beyond the simple appearance of things. This does not mean that the mask is not real, for it is. It's just that your eyes have been opened to the greater reality of the world by gaining the Second Sight, the vision granted by the forbidden ointments and magick of Faery. When this vision is gained what you might have very well assumed until then to be all there was of reality suddenly becomes but one small portion of it, just one layer of many.

Sadly, though, once that rush passes away, the memory you are left with cannot compare to all that you have learned and felt and experienced. When the door closes, we are left with a sad assortment of tools in which to remember it and try to express it to others, our family, friends, and fellow Witches. We're forced to fumble with words, trying to make them mean more, to express what is pretty near impossible to express. Our modern languages especially are not well suited to the task; they've become far too concretized to hold the magick and meaning of the ancient world of myth and poetry, of legend and of dream.

Not that it doesn't creep out now and then, appearing to us in quick flashes of insight and revelation, both in ritual and even in our books and movies. Books and movies which are, after all, gifts of the Muse and reflections of our own mythology. Unfortunately, we just don't expect it anymore, not like in the past. Poets and bards were once expected to speak with the voice of the Divine, much as oracles did, as well as Kings and Queens, Priests and Priestesses.

In the past, words were still credited with the power to work magick in poem and prayer, in chant and rune and song. The same sort of magick that a Witch could do, since both poet and Witch flirted with madness as they walked on the edge of the wild, upon the sword's blade bridge between this world and the world of Other. As they dared to peer into all the marvelous and terrifying worlds that lie in the beyond and learned to give expression to those visions here.

Doorways can still be formed by poetry, though, as by any other tool of the art. Though, as always, be careful what you ask for.

A Ritual to Start Upon the Path to The Beyond

Draw a circle and stand within it. Become aware of the boundaries of the circle, the boundaries of what is known. It is dark beyond the flame of your candles, but there are other lights out there. The flickering of possibilities and ideas and powers which have not found realization here upon the Earth, the tender sparks of that which as yet has no mask or form or face. All this lies in the beyond, gifts as yet unearned, unclaimed, unknown.

Become aware that there are many roads around you, roads that lead out into that darkness, which lead to those distant lights. Each road is different. No two journeys are the same. One road will appeal more to one person than another, though all of them have challenges that will have to be overcome. These challenges may be different on the outside, but they always involve a testing of self and of claiming who you are and of your own power and place in the universe.

Ask for a door to be opened.

Ask for your road to be shown to you, the road that is most proper for you to take.

Ask for guides and guardians, for companions and helpmeets. Keep your heart open towards who or what may show up to do that, for it is different for everyone. Do not judge who comes for another, for who knows what may come to your own aid.

Ask all of this out of love and in the hopes that you will become all that you were always meant to be. Knowing that in this way you will be able to walk once more in those distant lands, to reach those faraway lights, and to bring back to the Erth, back to your friends and family and to the whole human race what is most needed in this place and in this time.

The following words may be used, if desired:

I ask for a door
For a road
For a path
Be shown me
I ask for aid and comfort
Guides along the way
To be
To know

To do

To dare
And return once more.
Seven steps to take me there
And the eighth to bring
Me back again.

There are many paths and you will need to pick the one you wish most to walk, the one that calls out to you. Choice is action and choosing and doing are part of the perfecting of the nature when it comes to learning to be a Witch of the old ways, of the Old Ones. Not that it will be easy or safe. But when has that ever stopped a true Witch, a Witch of the heart?

Knot Charms

One, two, pluck a cord
A jangling sound a spell is born
It holds the form
It holds the name as well
For what is woven is in part of you
And part of what may be
Spiders all
We weave and are woven
Are called and sworn and bold to be
And so are known
And so must pass away
As dewdrops in a web
Glimmer and are gone

A spell of knots is a way to hold that which cannot otherwise be held such as a spirit, a thought, a dream, a spell. A knot was, of old, a form of a charm, a sort of binding. You breathed upon the cord, the thread, the plait, the rope, and the name of what you breathed, its essence, was captured in the knot you tied. The cord itself was already a weaving of sorts, for in olden days, spinning and weaving were arts within themselves, woman's magick. To weave and to create thread and cloth, tapestries and clothes—symbolic of the forms that we take on as spirits take on fleshly apparel—lay within the hands of Goddesses and spiders, a talent that they taught to but a select few.

Sailors know of this trick and bought cords of the winds from sorceresses, for Witches of the ancient times long had an accord with the fancies of the Air who allowed themselves to be captured and so held, if only for a time. When the ship found itself far out to sea and the sails would grow still, then a knot could be undone and a wind loosed to fill the canvas once more. Or, if you required even greater speed, you could undo two knots and let out two winds. Three knots were said to release a storm, which was not highly recommended.

As with all spirits of the Air, their magick lies in the breath itself, in the word, in a name and a cry, in the rising mist of sweet incense, in knowing how to laugh and realizing that you can fly. It exists in the whispering spirit lying cradled in your ear to tell you of what you otherwise could never know. It exists in the tales of the traveling wind, which goes far and returns again, bringing back mystery and knowledge and the scents of far off lands. It is a wind which cannot be stilled overlong, even in a knot which some sailor bought or that some Witch tied.

To Perform a Knot Charm

Take a length of cord or twine or thread and breathe upon it. Fix in your mind what it is you wish to keep and, having that firmly in your mind, tie the knot with the intent of capturing it within.

Kiss the knot and, as you do, concentrate upon the name and nature of that which you wish fixed to the thread. For this, you will need to be able to feel the essence of what you are putting into the knot for safekeeping, to feel it so very intensely that you have in some ways become the very thing which you are concentrating on. You have become a part of it, as it has become a part of you, just as the true name of a thing is also the thing itself. This kind of intense Knowing is key to many magicks of the past.

The following words may be used if so desired:

Fixed and found
In this cord abide
In this knot be bound
Til it be undone

But, again, be mindful that no knot can hold something for long, so that this is a spell which can only capture that which truly wishes to be captured and will only be held for a little while. Accordingly, this gift should be always be honored and used in a proper manner and never lightly.

Blessings

Ash and dust
Barley meal and blood
One long trickle of wine as red
As the seed which kept heaven chained
Pouring down as rain
Upswept mouths
Hungry for the pleasure
Of the divine
Longing so for love
And for a taste
Of what cannot bear to be denied.

It is a long tradition to bless food before eating it, to be thankful. But you should not just be thankful for the food, but have respect for the idea of reciprocity that it symbolizes. You give in order that more may be given, so that you may receive in turn, not out of a sense of entitlement or that of a bargain made—for you must give as freely as you receive, not expecting it—but simply knowing that this is the nature of the greater universe around you. Acknowledging and being thankful for food, as with any gift, helps keep the flow of energy going, helps keep the wheel turning.

You should also learn to eat the food that are needs, not necessarily just those which are desires. Desire and need are not the same thing, just as desire and bliss are not the same thing. Bliss is part of ones' self, of who and what you are. So what you eat and drink should lend itself to this, to a purification of the whole, body, mind, and spirit. You should eat and drink with an understanding of this process and what is proper for your self and body. You should bless the imparting of those virtues in what you are going to eat and drink, because in this way you also bless yourself.

In the past, when people grew their own food, they put their effort and intent into creating it for the purpose of the furtherance of life. They blessed the fields, blessed the crops, and blessed the bread. Every step from planting the seeds to sitting at the table to eat the finished loaf was acknowledged and seen as part of a greater whole. It symbolized an intimate connection between you and the land you lived on, and the Gods and the spirits of the land you lived with. The same holds true for blessing the trees which produce the nuts and fruit and blessing the grapes and vines which are needed to create the wine. All in understanding that to extend such blessings extends to you the same energy and love which comes from the source and returns to it once more.

The cornucopia or Horn of Plenty is a symbol of this cycle of endless bounty and abundance. It continually pours forth all good things, and that which pours forth takes shape according to what is needed. Fruits, grains, and even humankind itself. Goodness and purity of beauty, purity of self. The sort of purity which is to be the best and most of who and what you were born here to be, the shape you take upon the Earth in order to fulfill a particular need. All because we are also a part of the bounty and abundance of the earth. This is a power of the North and of the God of the North for it is both about Being and about life's eternal abundance.

But we don't just bless food to show we are thankful or to express our understanding of the cycle, but because blessing can also energize the food. Whatever enters the body becomes of it—as the saying goes, you are what you eat—so that you should consume that which is pure in order to become and remain pure. All food can be blessed, even a simple peanut butter and jelly sandwich. Good food makes a good body. Better food makes a better body, a strong foundation for the spirit inside to be able to shine.

At the very least, health issues distract you from more spiritual pursuits, though they can also serve to point a finger at not just physical blocks and wounds in our energies, but emotional and psychic ones. For we are all multiple beings, even as we are one being. We are as much made up of energies interacting with other energies as energy interacting with matter, especially since matter takes its cues from energy, the physical body from the spiritual aspect. We need to be in balance with the energies that flow through us as it also flows through the land around us, everything participating in the natural order. That is what it means to be a part of the

225

land, part of the cycle.

To bless is to remind what is being blessed of its continual and continued connection to life's source—to recall to it the shape it was meant to take, the purity of its essence. In this way, you eat and drink of the things of the divine. Every meal can and should be a sacrament, a thing made sacred, a ritual of joy and participation in life. It's an acknowledgement that the universe can and does provide if you have faith in it that it will, when deep down you know and believe it is a place of bounty and not a place of lack. We set our own table with our beliefs, so that it either holds a fEast as grand as might serve a king or nothing more than a beggar's poor portion of crumb and crust.

This thought can extend not just to the dinner table, but to other aspects of your life. To bless that which comes to you, to be thankful for it, opens yourself up to future gifts, to keeping you in the flow, keeping the circle going. However, to allow more to come into your life, sometimes you have to make room by getting rid of that which you honestly don't need. Getting rid of things can be a literal or a figurative act or both; it can be a very freeing and cleansing and it would be a good idea to do it at least once a year, more often if you find yourself confused or at odds with your life. What was no longer to your benefit may benefit others, which will come back to you in the long run.

Out with the old, in with the new—a literal and spiritual spring-cleaning is sometimes what we need most, and what we find it difficult to do. It's hard to give up things, especially when our culture teaches us that things are what we need to make ourselves happy. But you should sit back every now and then and take a good hard look at your life and decide what it is you really want, what it is that really makes you happy and fulfilled. Who are you really, what do you want to do, how can you get there, and what you can get rid of in order to lighten your load and make you free enough to follow your truth path, your greatest bliss.

However, in giving to others—whether actual physical things you've decided to clear out of your life, but that someone else can still get good use of—or thoughts or ideas or even services, you should always give as much as possible with no thought of return. Certainly, there should be no little tally book being kept in the back of your mind that says that since you gave *this*, you are now deserving of *that*. You have to just do it out of the simple joy of giving, of participating in the circle of prosperity, of taking an active part of the free flow of energy. Because doing it reluctantly, or with some sense of entitlement of return, attaches the wrong sort of energy to the act and can restrict the flow.

Give without expectation of control, without knowing or worrying about what the person receiving the gift will or will not do with it, because once it's out of your hands it's really no longer any of your concern. The more you do it, the easier this will become and with an ease of giving comes an ease of receiving, which for some is the more difficult lesson. If you can give to others with joy, with no expectation, but because you simply want to give...joy shall be your return. Gifts will come to you and doors will open, both within you and in the world at large.

Gifts are seeds. People used to bless the trees in order that they might blossom and fruit; they made offerings to them and gave to the Gods and the spirits of the fields. They gave back of part of each harvest so that the energies would pass onwards and kept some of the seeds each fall so that they could be planted the next spring, so that the trees and fields would bloom again. Today, even if we do not keep fruit trees or plant wheat or corn ourselves, we can still live the same metaphor in our lives by "feeding" the first fruits to our own Gods and spirits. By acknowledging the circle that we are all a part of.

A peanut butter and jelly sandwich, a cookie, a bright red apple in your hand, just the sort that gave rise to the myth of the fall of human nature, these are all gifts that should be acknowledged, just as any gift needs to be acknowledged and cherished. All the while, nor forgetting to give of yourself to friends and family in your life, to the whole around you, because each of us are also gifts.

Gobah...it is the circle that encompasses us all. I give so that you may give and so that I may give again. I give so that you may be more so that in your being more, I will be more. It is a living and vital link between us all, to give and to receive freely.

A Blessing for the Feast

This can be done in ritual or out of ritual, perhaps at a dinner shared by your coven. The Priest or Priestess can say the words, or everyone can say them together.

Bless this food—may it lend purity and strength to mind, body, spirit, and purpose.

It is part of the circle as we are part of the circle, and so to acknowledge the fEast is to acknowledge ourselves and all that we can be. Light and power grounded in the earth, we who bear the patterns of the stars to the world below, and who must never ever forget.

Bless this drink—may it lend purity and strength to mind, body, spirit, and purpose.

The gift of life, the gift of love, the gift of need, and the gift of clarity, may we all find it within our hearts, within our selves, within each other, so that we may seek it within the world around us, the world outside this, our own small circle.

So, to eat, to drink, to make merry in all we do and say, this is the best blessing of all.

Gobah.

Glamourie

It's not too much then to expect
For a Witch to transform to a shape of cat
Or for a cat to like to keep a Witch
By their whimsy, strictest rule, and wish
Such wayward spirits take the form
Of familiar flesh to bring them back
The mirror that keeps the candle's wake
Is also a door to other states

We are all spirits riding around within a tender vehicle of flesh. What is eternal is what lies within, but the flesh often comes to mirror the spirit. The body takes on the form that the soul dictates, dressed by years of emotions and thoughts and feelings and beliefs, both the good and the bad. The more closely you are in tune with your true spirit, the more closely your physical form can come to reflect that spirit. As it also influences what you broadcast to the world around you, for how people see us is a combination of our actual physical form and the impression of ourselves that we broadcast.

This is the source of the magick of the glamour or glamourie, an image sent out to beWitch or bewilder, to charm or to frighten. As Witches we can learn how to use the energies inside us to send out what we desire to send out, to influence how others perceive us. For example, when you meet someone you can often sense things about them, an impression that can even overlay their actual physical impression generated by what they look like, what they say and do. Normally, this is not under the conscious control of the person giving off the impression, but a Witch can learn to control what energies they send off and so how they come to be "seen" and remembered. This stems from having a strong connection to the spirit within, our own individual spark of light and life.

Despite the common thought that a glamourie is meant to confuse or deceive, the real goal of learning to consciously control this energy is not to twist or to cloak that light, but to embrace it as fully as possible. We are meant to let it shine through us, through our bodies, as directly as possible—as though your physical form was but a pane of glass and your spirit the sun shining through that glass. Still, the energy that we send out all around us is flavored not only by who we are deep inside, but also by what we think of ourselves. Unfortunately, this impression may not always be true or even all that good for us. It can too easily be influenced by what others think of us or want us to think of ourselves, and so be led astray from who we are really are. Especially since it is often easier to take on the aura of what others make us out to be, rather than who we are really meant to be.

What we send out into the world, what we broadcast about who we are, can have a profound effect, an effect that we can learn to harness. It is simple enough to become adept at broadcasting messages such as "leave me alone," "don't notice me," or "pay attention to me," in the right circumstances. "Come here" or "go away" broadcasts are the easiest of all and, quite often, instinctively sent. But when you get control over what you broadcast, you can send out stronger and more complex messages, learning to cloak yourself in glamour, shadow, and seemings.

The trick is that this seeming comes from someplace deep inside you, so that in a fashion you have convince *yourself* of the reality of it in order to be able to best project that reality to those around you. You have to know that what you are broadcasting is "true;" the more you believe this, the more powerful the glamour will be. This is similar to the thought that the best liars as those who believe their own lies, who strongly believe in the false world that they have created.

The hard part lies in convincing your deepest self, your subconscious, to believe that something is absolutely true, while, at the same time, keeping in mind that what you are seeking to convince it of *isn't* absolutely true—so that you don't end up convincing your own self of a false reality. For example, if you broadcast that you are someone of no importance, in seeking not to be noticed, you must be careful not to have it backlash into your own psyche, so that you begin to believe you are not important.

As a glamour is a projection, an illusion, so the stronger the belief in it, the stronger the illusion. You are projecting into someone else's awareness that you look like a cat or a bird or someone else, or that you are taller or scarier or have a different eye or hair color. Though to *actually* transform physically takes an even stronger belief and the ability to be able to sidestep into another world, a word where such transformation is not only possible, but even easy. For the body takes it cues from the spirit and the power of the spirit springs from faith. Faith, which is also known as fate…

So, to alter your fate, as in that which this life desired you to be—a man, a woman, a human being or a cat, taller, shorter, whatever—you must alter your faith in as absolute a manner as possible. In this, doubt becomes your biggest obstacle, doubt and an engrained faith in the rules created by the modern science and society. Though science has begun at the last to dabble in realms that might be considered mystical, and there to "discover" oddities and truths that others have long known about, its old rules still hold sway over most of us today. Rules which include an absolute denial of the ability of anyone to actually and physically alter their shape.

In order to get past this great wall of doubt, you have to start simple. You have to work on gaining the power of the glamour before working your way up to attempting what lies beyond it. You need to polish your abilities of illusion, before playing around with changing reality itself. Of course, this sort of spell can also reveal that which you may not wish revealed—as your own fears and problems may become projected around you—so self-awareness is a must.

To be honest, a lifetime of study and practice might not prove enough to gain again the power of shapeshifting, not with all the stumbling blocks set in our way. But, one never knows, miracles can and do happen all the time. This power was well known to the Old Ones, the Witches of the past, and no power ever known can be entirely lost again. It may take generations to come, Witches raised with the belief that it is possible rather than impossible, in order to get back to that ability. But if we desire it strongly enough and need it, the power can and will return to us.

A Charm of Glamour

First off, you have to get a grip on what you are already projecting to the world around you. Ask yourself, what do you believe, deep down, about yourself, and also go to your friends and family and ask them how they see you. Bearing in mind, of course, that how they see can also be influenced by their own projections.

Experiment with going to parties or out in public and try to alter what you are broadcasting. If you are normally shy, try to send out feelings that you are approachable and friendly. If you are normally very gregarious, try to broadcast that you are shy. Try to get people to see you as older or younger by taking on yourself a feeling that you are a different age than you really are. Of course, you can help with that illusion by dressing to suit the age you want to project. Just as there are many color choices that can help you broadcast a different feeling, whether one of peacefulness or aggression.

Like any other skill, it takes time and practice. You have to first learn how to sense the energy that you are projecting, before you can learn to control it. When you control what you are sending out, only then you will be able to influence how others perceive you.

Some words you can use:

May what is within
Be seen without
Work this magick
Around and about
What I believe
Is what you see.

To Connect to the Fey

They watch with foxes' eyes,
Green ivy night flower
They peer around the trunk of the great oak tree
High on the bluff
Where the river runs and makes a boundary
With the world of mists and dreams.
Broken shards of pottery is all that remains
Of those who once knew their call
They are not foxes
But they think like one,
Quick and sharp as a knife of flint
And bone

This is a true story. It's a story of ghost fog and of the distant glow of a fire where those we had just celebrated our rituals with were now gathered around to talk and drink and make merry in whatever way took their fancy. We could have been with them, enjoying the fire and the company, the mead and wine and laughter. But instead, one by one, we drifted away from the light and walked into the night. It was chilly and a mist had risen from the ground, shrouding the trees, and making the woods mysterious and haunted, as though they were not the same woods they had been by day. A full moon gleamed through the mist and fog, turning everything tarnished silver.

We followed a narrow path, feeling the chill settle deeper into our bones as we walked, a chill which wasn't entirely due to the temperature. It was as if the modern world fell away the deeper we went into the woods, into the darkness. The path led us to what remained of an old building, though all that was left was an old stone foundation and a partially tumbled-down hearth. The hearth stood to the South, perfect to hold and symbolize the power of Fire.

We lit candles. One, two, three, four, tiny sparks of light in the dark, one for each Quarter. A circle was measured out by steady tread. The trees seemed to gather closer still, darkness like a cloak between them, the moon riding high above. No one could see us now. We had gone elsewhere, deeper into the night and the past and into the forms of mystery.

Our candles seemed dim protection against anything beyond our tiny circle. But then they were not meant to protect, but to call. As we all shivered with the chill, one woman stepped forward and spoke to the East. Old words rang out, a command and a call, weaving the beginnings of an ancient spell, a beautiful bargain, the memory of what was and what would be again.

And we were suddenly not alone.

The darkness between the trees held figures now, tall, thin, pale figures with drifting arms and huge black eyes. Some of us could only sense their presence, but a few of us could actually see them, peering around the trunks of trees. We knew them as they knew us. How could we have forgotten the pure darkness of those perfectly shaped eyes, the almost translucent glow of their skin, the floating elegance of their long arms and long fingers. We felt both frightened and reassured as they peered at us from out of the shadows, from behind doors in the very fabric of reality.

Tonight was their night. Tonight was our night. Tonight, we would reach out to each other across worlds, and rebuild what was to carry us into what was, and what might be again. One by one, we were brought forward to face the Eastern edge of the circle and there to meet our match, the one who had come there just for us, the one who loved us best of all. And there in the dark, in the mist, by the moonlight, we were bound together once again. Not that we had ever truly been apart, except that we were the ones who had forgotten the Other and this night would now remind us of just what we had forgotten.

For most of us have forgotten not just who we are, but that we are of a shared nature. That who and what we truly are lies inside us, waiting to be awakened, to be acknowledged—who we are and where we came from, and why these tall pale folk of the Air are our brothers and sisters, as much as those who had remained by the fire this evening. One breath, two, the cold unacknowledged now as we stood in their company, as we stood in the fringes of the Otherworld. As we became one once more, together in the circle with our reclaimed friends and companions, our long lost family.

For those that time and legend and storytales have come to call the Fey, the Faery, the gentry, the Shining Ones, have always been with us, a part of our lives and love and fate. They have an old and intimate connection with Witches, with those of the Blood. Together with the Fey, we share the history of the Earth and of the stars, just as we share in the responsibility of being guardians and guides and healers and teachers to all who live here. They are those who watch, in whose charge is the great work that is in progress here upon the earth, the unfolding of the plan that we are all an intimate part of.

They are many and one. Individual, yet capable of speaking and acting as one. Spirits of the wind and of the air, of breath and boundless spirit. Spirits who laugh above all other things, to laugh for the boundless beauty and joy of it all.

But they can speak for themselves:

We are not small spirits. There are spirits for all things in nature, for all that lives has its spiritual echo. Spirits of a natural world and even of places, but we who are of the air and those who are of the water, we are those of whom the fairytale is told. We are the hosts—as you are the guests—and they of the waters are the rushing horde. We are all of air as they are all of water, while they who are earth and they who are fire you will not find in the old tales, not in the guise of they who you now name "Faery."

See us, if you wish, as small slender things with wings, as pixies, aliens, elves, and the other shapes your imagination paints us with, but know it is you who give us form. What remains true to us is the whirl of the wind, whiteness, the withy glow, and the black of a sharp eye, which is, in itself, a symbol. As for they of the waters—to rush, to run, greyness, never only one, and the black of the perfect round. All the rest is but dream and desire.

We are the first ones, the Elder Children, we who were born before the world began. Time is a new invention to us, still a plaything. A spinning top. A hall of mirrors.

We step in and out of what you call existence, yet what you see is only half of what is. We live in the other half. But we return again and again to the world of sight, for many are our families there. And we are much in love with flesh. It calls to us, beautiful physicality. Pain and pleasures are but sensations, and all the senses are creations of art and majesty. Without them, the Divine is blind, dumb, shriven and alone.

See each other, know each other, touch each other—it is what you are here for. It is why we are born back to flesh. There is no tomorrow that is also not yesterday and so we are your ancestors and yet your children. We love you. We are you. The first shall be last and the last shall be first. This is the riddle of the illusion of time, and of our own existence in eternity.

We are the Elder Children and you the younger. But yet the first shall be last, and the world was born in one day. A day that has not yet ended, and never shall.

So it is that we were not alone that night, and we are not alone in this world. We have never been alone. Spirits exist all around us, spirits of Earth, of Air, of Fire and of Water. Some of them are closer to us, more knowable because they think and feel and act in ways at least partially recognizable to us. But others are far more "alien," more strange and harder to understand.

The gentry and rushing horde—Faery folk, both—are two kinds of spirits long linked to Witches. One is of the East, of the Air, and one of the West and of Water. Of the two, the beings of Air are much nearer to us and have enjoyed a long and close relationship with those of the Blood. They have had many names throughout our history, but they are the source of the tales of the high court of the Seelie Sidhe, of the elves of light, and even of aliens who "abduct" poor unsuspecting human beings and take them to their flying saucers, just as the fair folk of old took other poor unsuspecting human beings to their fairy mound beneath the hollow hills. They who ride out on certain times of the year in grand procession, shining with their own light as they parade through woodlands and dance within the glades.

We have long known them as they have long known us. How we see them stems in part from our own expectations and from the stories of our own times, both conscious and unconscious, and so they become elves, a shining court, aliens, or even a giant insect which looks like some kind of praying mantis. Our own mind clothes them, overlying their essence with different forms. But, beneath it all, they remain the same. They who are named and perceived as elves, aliens, the Fey, the Sidhe, pixies, whirlwinds, who are the elemental spirits of the Air.

It is no coincidence that Witch and Faery have a long association; they are as close to Witchkind as brothers and sisters may be, and share the same path with us. Even though their own language is not our language and we cannot speak as they do, yet they can speak to us for they understand all tongues both ancient and modern. Just as they understand the language of symbols and of how to reach directly into the human heart and soul in order to be heard.

There is a Faery for every Witch, one who knows that Witch intimately and loves them most dearly. They are each in their own way a match for that Witch, a reflection of who and what they are, a mirrored opposite which meshes with the Witch's own feelings, strengths, weaknesses, fears, hopes, dreams, and beauty. When the gate is opened and the connection is made, a male Witch finds a female Faery greeting him from through the shimmering veil, while a female Witch is enfolded by a male Faery.

The Faery responds to the Witch by giving them a way to best touch that which they desire to find within themselves and so can be friend, companion, guide, lover, chastiser, consoler, brother, sister. They are yin to our yang, yang to our yin. While to the specific Faery, their Witch is the most fascinating and most precious being upon all the wide earth.

Their eyes, those deep, dark endlessly mysterious eyes, look upon us and see us as no other ever could. They look upon us with the eyes of profound and boundless love.

A Ritual to Acknowledge the Fey

In order to renew our friendship, to reclaim our ties of family with the Fey, it is a good idea to invite them to an earthly feast. Milk and cakes, especially round cakes, golden cakes made with honey, are good gifts to make. Fresh whole milk or even cream should be used, if possible. Just as the best cakes, are those which you have baked yourself. Wine may also be offered, red wine being the better choice.

The time to set out the feast is near or after midnight if at all possible. The best time of year is between May Day and All Hallows, though the best particular day is the Eve of All Hallows, when the veil between our world and theirs is at its thinnest.

You can choose to have a particular bowl or plate set aside to make your offerings if you want, white or green being the most appropriate colors. Something that won't break if you can leave it outside for the night might be a good idea. Though, if you don't live in a place where you can leave out bowls or plates of food or milk, then you can pick a particular spot close to home, such as the base of certain tree—and oak or ash or willow are all good choices.

Raise your bowl or plate and say out loud or silently:

All this I give freely
By earth and air
By fire and water
By all that is love
Sahmak hurralyia arahnak
Arahnak fama

Leave your bowl or plate there or pour it out at the base of the tree. Sometimes, you may find a gift will be given to you in return, or friendly tricks will be played on you to make sure that you know they are around and paying attention to you. More than one spare set of keys has gone missing, only to be found weeks later in the freezer of all places. It's just their kind of little joke. While a nicely woven basket once appeared in exchange for an item that the Fey appropriated for themselves.

If an item does disappear and you can't find it anywhere, no matter how hard you've looked, you can ask nicely for them to return it. Afterwards, looking in the same places that you've previously looked before will often find it there in plain sight.

The power of the Fey is laughter, and their magicks are based upon laughter. A laughter which springs from the inner workings of the universe itself.

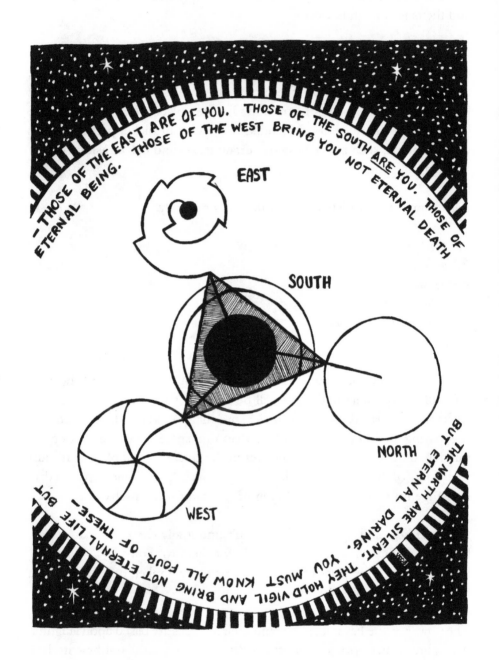

Part Four
Elements and Pathways

Once men hunted a ghost in the dark, a white stag, pure as snow. Pure as they longed in their hearts to be.

But even the white stag bleeds red, and red is the color of courage, of sacrifice, of desire.

The color of Kingship is not purple, but red. For their blood is the blood of the stag and so they wear a crown of antlers, knowing they and the hunted were once brothers.

Kings were crowned upon the great hills, for the great hills were the first watchtowers. The boundaries are defined not by one thing, but by four. For that is the way of it. The watchtowers are twofold and, hence, fourfold as well. As any good king.

A King is known by his crown, his blood, his wand, his heart.

A King's crown is the weight of responsibility and remembrance, the blood which binds him to land and kin, the wand to create fruit and grain for the hungry and the lost, and his heart to forgive those who transgress against him.

A Queen is known by her love, her light, her cup, her garter.

The love enfolding of all, the light illuminating the darkest places, the cup so that all may drink and know and remember, and the garter to recall the days when even Gods walked among us

The true throne that they share is one of stone and of flesh. In a kiss all is shared.

The sons of royalty are the Four Quarters of the Earth, the center of which bears the hill where the sky meets the shores of earth.

And all begins again.

The Wheel

Witch power is phoenix power—life, death, rebirth, endless and everlasting transformation.

Love is the power of the soul making itself known. Love is, more than anything else, and so love becomes whenever there is need of it. What was lost is found again; such is the way of things and always has been.

For we are children of the stars and of the patterns of the heavens and so those patterns resound in our souls, in our hearts, and when we walk them we recall not only our true origins, but our very selves. We are children of the Fire of the Gods and so it lives within the vehicle of our Blood, waiting for those patterns to rouse it back to full force. We are the children of the wheel of time, whose goal is not to remove ourselves from it, but to transcend it.

We are the children of love, which is the phoenix.

There are eight Sabbats and each one of them corresponds to one of the four Quarters or the four Cross-Quarters. There are also four Gates, the Gates of North and South and East and West. The pillars stand at the Cross Quarters, whose powers are only called upon for need.

North is Midsummer and equates to Earth.
North-East is May Day and equates to Earth and Air.
East is Spring Equinox and equates to Air.
South-East is Imbolc and equates to Air and Fire.
South is Yule and equates to Fire.
South-West is All Hallows and equates to Fire and Water.
West is Autumn Equinox and equates to Water.
North-West is Lammas and equates to Water and Earth.

Note: The above Sabbat names are used here for reference only as they have other names in the old Witch language.

242

The Four Elements are Earth, Air, Fire, and Water.

The Eight Elements are Earth, Soot, Air, Sulphur, Fire, Blood, Water, and Clay.

The Four Essences are Being, Knowing, Doing, and Daring.

The Eight Essences are Being, Traveling, Knowing, Teaching, Doing, Ecstasy, Daring, and Making.

North is Earth and noon and Midsummer, both the height of the day and the height of the season. This is the time of the Goddess of the North, Ardwena, and her most beloved South God, Tzahranos. It is the time of life and light, of fertility of body, mind, and spirit. It is the day of Earth and of action. At Midsummer we reach the full glory of the summer season, which was begun at May Day and which shall ebb into Lammas.

South is midnight, the silent waiting cave, Midwinter. Here we find the North God, Eahnos, the silent one Himself, and the South Goddess of Priestesses through all time, Sahlonshai. It is the time of silence and of Fire, of giving birth to fire within the darkness of the cave, the darkness of self. This is the high tide of winter, which began at All Hallows and shall change again at Imbolc.

East is dawn and the pale and glimmering star road of the Spring Equinox, the white buds that will blossom into the flowers of May. The Queen of Elphame, Arien, is the East Goddess and with Her, the God of the West, Hehren. Air and Daring are both required in order to proceed from this point. This is the high tide of spring which began at Imbolc and shall close at May Day.

West is dusk, Fall Equinox, and the time of harvest and of willing sacrifice to make the seeds of tomorrow. This is the time of Ariadne, the Goddess of the West, of Water and of inspiration. The waters of inspiration and the sacrifice needed in order to feed what is given. It is also the time of Tehot, the God of the East and of knowledge. This is the high point of the autumn, which started at Lammas and shall end at All Hallows.

These are the Sabbats of the Solstices and Equinoxes, while the Cross-Quarter Sabbats are May Day, Imbolc, All Hallows, and Lammas.

May Day lies between Air and Earth and is the time of traveling, of going to the Otherworld as those of the Otherworld came to us at the Sabbat that faces it across the wheel, All Hallows. Whatever fEast and whatever welcome we tendered to them at that time returns to us at in May, so it is not just to your credit, but to your benefit to be generous and kind. Gehhest is here, the God of travelers, the guide to the place of the Good Game.

Imbolc lies between Air and Fire and is when the powers of illumination are called upon, the fires which once danced upon the heads of the apostles in the Christian faith and made them able to understand and speak all languages, including the language of the heart. This is the Sabbat of spiritual re-birth, a birth of understanding. Ahtamenak is the God of Imbolc and Gwenhyvar the Goddess, both of them teachers in their own way.

All Hallows stands between Fire and Water and is when—as most people know—the veil is thin between this world and the Otherworld. But the veil is not just thin at this time with only the realm of the dead and the realm of Faery, but with all other worlds and all other realms. At this sacred time, magick crosses all boundaries easier and can have far-reaching consequences as a result. It is also the start of the year, for the time between All Hallows and Midwinter is the dead time, the fallow time, when one should rest and reflect. All Hallows is the Sabbat of Morgah and Akenahmnos, Goddess and God of ecstasy and transformation, of life and death intermingled in love.

Lammas is the place where Earth meets Water and it is the most unknowable to us as they are both eternal powers, unlike Fire and Air. This is where physical form and life is created, as Fire and Air come together at Imbolc to bring the spark of the divine and the breath of spirit. This is where we ask that the land and the waters provide for the continuation of life, to give us what we most need in order to survive. Lammas is the time of Hekahteh and Ahdtar, both of whom understand the making of things whether through the clay of the body or the shape of a spell.

As the Wheel turns, the powers ebb and flow, each season passing into the next, each year, each Age. The powers preside over different times of the year, as the Wheel goes from the dark into the light and back into the dark once more, as we pass from life into death and back to life again, a count of beads upon an eternal necklace. In this way, you can look at each Sabbat as an individual event, but to truly understand them you have to look at the whole that they create together.

As we celebrate the Sabbats, we celebrate the pattern that the Sabbats make. They are a part of our own inner landscape, as much as the seasons, the pillars and the gates. As we learn about them, we learn about ourselves. As we follow the pattern, we journey. We call upon the powers within and the powers without—powers that share in and reflect each other's natures—so that when we are grounded and centered within the foundation and central point of our highest, our best self, we become our own wellspring of power. We become the center of that turning Wheel, the spark from which the beams of light pour forth in four directions, in eight, in sixteen.

The Wheel is the same symbol as the shimmering halo of the *sained* ones, the holy ones, mighty and pure, and all of this lives inside us, sleeps inside us, waiting to be acknowledged, welcomed, and released. It waits for us to become mirrors for our own souls, windows for the blessing of divine providence. We can become prisms and crystals, through which the eternal light can shine and bring beauty and grace and love to the earth and to each other.

By celebrating the Sabbats in turn, we undertake a journey to discover that inner light. We discover ourselves and open our hearts, allowing it to become the central point of the Wheel, allowing the powers the form the directions and the seasons to flow through us. You can take this journey many, many times and yet it will always have something new to show you, something amazing to teach you.

Not surprisingly, the spokes of the Wheel can also been seen as being roads. Roads that, to travel upon them to the very end, would find you returning once again though their opposite. For example, if the road that you choose to take is the way of the South-East—of Air and Fire, of illumination and sacrifice—then you will eventually return through the door of the North-West, the door of Earth and Water, of silence and of the making of things.

By exploring these roads, the Gods and the Sabbats and the gates, we can come to the light that shines at the center of all. It is a beautiful thing, breathless and freeing, peaceful and yet filling you up with the desire to go and move and do, to act both in and out of this world. When you find this light and let it into your heart, you feel fully alive and aware as never before and you find your balance. And once you have experienced this, you will not forget it, nor wish to give it up again.

People search their whole lives for what is already around them, for what is already inside of them. This is in part of because of the limited ways of seeing that we are taught by science and most modern religions. For example, when you view time in only one way, as linear rather than circular, as a straight line rather than a Wheel, you limit yourself and you limit this world. Just as believing that only what can be seen with the naked eye or under a microscope—only what science can "prove" exists—is all there is limits you to a very small and rather shallow universe.

When you find the center, you can see all and you will know the peace of the eternal. Not the peace of doing nothing, of withdrawal from the world like some monk or hermit, but the peace that lies where the spokes of the Wheel come together as one, the place where you and your life is in perfect accord. It is in this state of mind and being that you will know why you are here and what your place in the world is. It is here that the bright fire fills you up and makes you a Shining One. As you become a doorway for the powers that exist out there in the Great Unknown.

As all the elements and essences are associated with and symbolized by various of the Gods and Goddesses, each according to Their own nature, the same can be said for each Witch, every one of the *Sorgitza*. As with the Gods, we are living masks for powers, elements, and essences larger than ourselves. We are here, in part, much as windows or crystals, mirrors and gates, in order to project and channel those powers into the material world.

To see beyond the world of form is to see into other worlds. To look past the mere appearance of things is the Second Sight, a means of seeing which stems from the heart and not from the eyes. The Second Sight is a key towards unlocking the ability to affect these other worlds, the Unseen realms, and by extension and reflection this world. It is also key in forming deep relationships with the spirits and beings who are the living and conscious masks of the essences and elements. The Second Sight reveals what lies beneath the skin of the world, allowing you to begin working more directly with the greater powers.

We need these living masks for few of us can long bear the naked face of the Divine, an essence which is ultimately unknowable in its entirety. In fact, the closer that we get to catching a glimpse of that ultimate, the more paradoxical and alien to us become the powers and beings that we must interact with. This is why the Gods and Goddesses that we are more inclined to form relationships with are the smaller or lesser Gods, those who yet retain an understanding and concern for our problems, needs, and desires here in the world. Still, through interaction with these lesser Gods, through learning from Them and forming relationships with Them, we can in turn grasp at greater and ever greater Gods. This will, eventually, lead us all the way back to the Source itself.

Our physical bodies are not really built at this time to hold onto the essence of the greater powers for long periods of time, at least not without years and years of training and purification. In particular, it is very important that you have a good, strong foundation of self when you wish to take up the challenge, so that you will not prove lesser than that which you have called up and end up risking having it overwhelm you.

You must be balanced in mind, body, and spirit in order to let that kind of power through and not possibly be hurt by it, emotionally or physically. It's for this reason that Witches go through tests and are reborn physically and spiritually as "other," so that they can stand with a foot in two different worlds and better withstand the energies that they work with and channel. Energies that otherwise would be too difficult or dangerous to handle. Though there is always a risk, even for an experienced Witch.

There are Seen and Unseen powers. The Seen powers are the elements of Earth, Air, Fire, and Water, while the Unseen sides of the elements are Being, Knowing, Doing, and Daring. These powers come together as roads and form the crossroads, which is the traditional meeting place of Witches. Of old, Witches met not necessarily at a literal crossroads, but at the crossroads of the four Elements. They met at the point where the four came together as one and formed a foundation of boundless possibility. An elemental crossroads, which also exists inside each Witch, giving each of us our own foundation for the temple of self.

We are made of all four Elements. The moon is our Mother and the Earth is our Mother, one being the Goddess of our bodies and the other the Goddess of our souls. Just as the sun is our Father and the living water is our Father, one being the God of our bodies and the other the God of our spirits. From Water and Earth we are formed, but what moves us is Fire and Air, breath and the spark of life. In this way, we are as much made of the four Elements as the rest of creation, just as we are made up of the interplay of the God and the Goddess.

Humankind sprang from clay, from Earth and Water, dust and blood. But blood is not just water, for the spark of Fire has been invested in it, making it truly alive, from which we get the old saying "the blood is the life." Blood is the medium for what moves us, for what makes us living. Blood is used in many rituals because it *is* the essence of life and magick; it holds the power of connection and of creation. It is Fire and Water intermingled, the South-West quarter. All blood does this, but Witch Blood even more so because it is conscious in its own right.

When the Blood is stirred up, it experiences both ecstasy and transformation, which is found in the Cross-Quarter of the South-West. This transformation can lead to greater and greater change, even to the ability to physically shapeshift. This change comes through the change in the consciousness of the Blood, that which is the true essence of the Witch. What the Blood believes becomes reality, as the flesh learns to take its cue from the spirit.

The South-East is teaching or bringing that which is within without, and sulphur, which represents the flame of knowledge. Sulphur is representative of the breath which is living spirit, breath which is the song and breath which is the word. When you combine Fire with Air you get illumination, the power that was "stolen" from the Gods, the power which "fell" from the heavens. This sort of illumination is a bright force of knowledge which is not learned but just *known*. This is the light which shines in all the dark places and wakes the powers that reside within us. Powers that, in a Witch, can be awoken by the dance, which connects us to the Old Ones and to our heritage.

But why is it sulphur? Poisonous gases were once used to open the mind, thus creating the ability to divine the future. Oracles would breathe in the fumes and lose themselves in the smoke, leaving their bodies to become doorways for the voice of Gods, Goddesses, and other spirits. It made them vessels for the powers of prophecy. Sulphur or brimstone creates a blue flame and its sweet sour smell has also long been associated with both

Witches and "the devil." It is the alchemy of Fire and of spirit, which firmly places it in the context of the South-East.

As the Fire of Water is blood and the Fire of Air is illumination so the Water of Earth is clay. Clay can be shaped and molded into many different forms. It is the most physically solid of all the elements and the oldest. To understand the North-West goes deeper than words. You have to go back into the world of instinct, of the memories that live within the body itself. Memories that were born when we first came into being, when we lived as one with our Mother, the Earth.

It is easy to see why clay and making would go together in the North-West, but what of soot and traveling in the North-East Quarter? The clue to this can be found in the Witch stories of the Middle Ages, where they were known to go to their rituals by flying up the chimney, the path of soot, of Earth and of Air. Soot was also mixed into the oils and ointments they once wore, which were also for "flying" or traveling. Not only did this mixture physically protect you from the cold, but the heat of your body activated the herbs and helped you achieve altered states of consciousness.

The elements of the Quarters and of the Cross-Quarters have an intimate relationship with each other, one represented by the interaction of the God and Goddess of that element, of the male and of the female essence that They symbolize. In the Quarters, the Goddess is the physical element— Earth, Air, Fire, or Water—and the God the metaphysical. In the Cross-Quarters, this is reversed and the Goddess is the metaphysical, while the God becomes the physical component of Soot, Sulphur, Blood, or Clay. But Cross-Quarter powers are not called in order to build essence, in order to set a foundation in place as with those of the four Quarters. The Cross-Quarters are only called up for need and for need alone.

As Ariadne, the Goddess of the West, tells us there are "*two guardians at each...black and white, male and female...the pillars are at the cross-quarters...the quarters hold the light and pillars there would block the light...*" The symbol of this is expressed by having a God and a Goddess for each—thus representing the dynamic polarity of male and female, black and white, past and future, all of the symbols of two that come together as one to form a greater whole.

Accordingly, to the South-East, the God of illumination stands back to back with the Goddess of the Quest. The God of the ecstasy of the Blood stands back to back with the Goddess of the hunt in the South-West. The God of the bEasts and wildwoods stands back to back with the Goddess of mysteries and secrets in the North-West. While, the God of the open gate takes one on the sword bridge to the Otherworld, to the field of roses, to the Game of Benevento in the North-East.

But each Quarter of the crossroads is also a road and forms a doorway to other realms. Accordingly, in the West, you will find the Gate of the Realm of the Dead. To pass through this Gate is to pass through the land of death and to what lies beyond. While, to the East, exists the Gate of the Realm of Faery. To explore past this Gate you must walk through the land of Faery. To the South, you will find the Gate of the Realm of the Stars, so named for the sparks of fire and light which once fell to the earth. And, finally, to the North, you will discover the Gate of the Realm of the Gods.

Each Gate has its own key, its own lesson to learn; you must find this key and learn this lesson in order to go through that door and enter its realm. Some will choose but to explore but one gate, one path, while others might pick one or two to learn, and this was often done in the past. But, for the coming time, the Gods have indicated that it would be better to find all four keys and to unlock all four gates yourself, gates which lie both within and without.

How we do this is by learning about the powers through interaction with them, through forming relationships with the beings and the Gods and Goddesses of the Elements. We learn about the powers by our enacting of the pattern of the Sabbats, the mask of the year. This is whywe celebrate at the Full Moons, because the moon is the lamp of night, that which is carried deep into darkness in order to discover the secrets hidden there, secrets which cannot be taught, but can only be felt. To dance beneath the full moon is to return to the beginning, to recall how the universe first came into being. It awakens the power of the Earth in our veins and our spirits soar, rising up in a beacon of light and power, reminding us that our nature is shared with the bright stars of the night sky

We come together to create a beacon which calls the old powers to us, powers of which we are a part. As our circles condense down to a single spark and at the same time expand out to enfold the entire universe. For to go out is to go in, and to go in is to go out. So the rim is the same as the center and the center is the same as the rim. We walk the roads and explore their dual nature—not just four, but eight, and not just eight, but sixteen—and as the Sabbats come into play one after the other each power builds upon the next, turning the Wheel. Until, at last, the pattern is closed and the spell complete, the spell of the year.

Watchtowers, gates, roads, pillars, Gods and Goddesses, in this way the Elements are represented, forming living masks for the powers that lie beyond them. By interaction with these masks, we interact with the Unseen world, which interlocks with our own visible earth. By interacting with them we celebrate the Wheel that forms the year, that sets the patterns upon the world and upon our hearts, and we go on the journey that is required of all.

Our Earthly Kin

The forest she waits for the touch of her kin
Known long ago, oh dread Ardwin
When the fires once burned in turn with the dark
Stars hung above where the bear left her mark
Deep in the stone, in the cup, in the bone
Of the earth, the great bEast, she struggles, is born
To reclaim the place of power and form
In the heart of her children from whom she was torn

To begin in the North is to begin in the place of Being, to have a strong and enduring connection to the Earth and to who you are. We need a good foundation as an individual and as a people, because without a good foundation we cannot go further without risking losing ourselves. Without a good strong foundation we can find ourselves at the mercy of the winds, to the storms of change, without anything to hold onto.

The North is the essence of strength, of surety, because the North is about Being, pure Being. This is a kind of Being that doesn't depend on you thinking anything or doing anything; it is about the silence and calmness that reside in the Earth and when we just *are*. It is a peace of the body, when you are in tune with what your body needs and with the rhythms and cycles that it is a part of.

As we are spirits who reside in bodies made of clay, made of the dust of the Earth, so each part of the Earth has its own spirit. The energy of a place is its living spirit, and as each place is different—from desert to mountain to plains to wetlands—so the spirits which exist in that land have different perspectives and personalities. When you move from one place to another, especially from one region to another, you enter into the realm of a new spirit. And when you have made a connection to the land

and the spirit of the land in one particular place, when you go to live in another place, you have to give up claim to the old and renew yourself in the new. You have to build a fresh connection to the land and to the spirits of the land.

To get to know the land you have to get to know its spirits. You have to be accepted by and form a bond with the consciousness of the land, especially with the overriding Earth spirit that has guardianship of that particular area. For through the Earth spirits reside everywhere, there are particular spots which contain a greater Earth spirit, one which commands the flow of energies that some call ley lines. The places that these greater spirits look out over tend to be the nexus points of the ley line energies, or the wellsprings from which the energies of the Earth emerge. These wellsprings, as previously indicated, tend to be sacred rivers or holy mountains.

The areas that are under the auspices and guardianship of the great Earth spirits are almost like kingdoms, and when you have pledged yourself to one you cannot go and then pledge yourself to another at the same time. In all politeness, when you travel from one region to another, you should ask the guardian spirit of the region you are visiting if it is all right that you enter its land. After all, you are about to be the guest of another country or kingdom. Permission is more than likely to be given, especially if you ask politely and honestly, and even if the spirit in question won't really be angry with you if you *don't* ask, it's still the proper thing to do. It shows proper respect if nothing else.

This doesn't mean that you can't move from one place to another, simply that once you've formed a connection to the land you shouldn't jump to another lightly or frivolously. For instance, the wellspring of the MidWest resides in the Black Hills of South Dakota, while if you cross the Mississippi—a boundary river—you will find yourself in the flow of power that stems from the Appalachians. If you live in one side of the river and connect to a spirit there, it will not be a light thing then to move to the opposite side and try to form a relationship. It can be done, but if you want a deep and strong connection, a good and lasting relationship, it takes time and commitment.

Years ago, we once contacted a guardian spirit of the land. At that time, we didn't really understand what it is we were interacting with. We were camping on the Western banks of the Mississippi river and, while out hiking around, we found an ancient mound and went and stood on top of it and tried to feel the energies inside it. It was a beautiful day with a pure blue sky overhead, the river flowing serenely Southward far below the bluffs we stood on. A large oak tree, hundreds of years old, had grown out of one side of the mound and its leaves rustled softly in the wind. Suddenly, we didn't feel alone and then something stirred beneath our feet, something huge and old and strong, something that was restless in its sleep.

It didn't wake up, not exactly, but it spoke to us and asked us who we were. It didn't understand how we could be there and yet not be connected to the ground we stood on. This didn't make any sense to it because the last time it had been awake the people who lived there had been different and they *had* an ancient connection to the Earth they lived with. We couldn't really answer the questions, in part because we didn't know ourselves what was missing from our lives, from our connection to the land. But this contact, even if fleeting, gave us a place to start.

It'd been scary to talk to something as old and powerful as that spirit, especially knowing that it hadn't even been fully awake the whole time it interacted with us. We felt the lingering effects of that contact for the rest of the evening and into the next day. But, it was years later that the events of that afternoon would take effect, when we were called upon by the Gods to wake up the spirits, to sing them from their sleep. It wasn't just the local spirits that woke, but that ancient spirit overlooking the Mississippi, a spirit hundreds of miles from where we lived and in another "kingdom."

Back in our own region, we began to court a connection to the spirit of that area, one that had not been asleep over the years. As we were directed by the Goddess of the North, the Goddess of Earth, we spoke to this spirit and gave it gifts and walked a labyrinth marked out in the grass. We walked it by day and sat in the center of it, feeling ourselves sinking downwards into the ground. And we walked it in the dark, by the flickering light of four torches, and felt an answering feeling stirring deep inside us. Each year, as we went to this place, we touched it and it touched us back, and ever so slowly a connection began to come into being, a relationship built on trust and honor and faith.

That first year, we held hands and formed a ring, watching as a bald eagle flew over our heads, circling three times before flying off towards the West.

We felt the Earth stir and whisper beneath our feet and what it might be like to belong once again, to belong after so long. Sometimes, the trees rustled in answer to our questions, their leaves moving even though there was no wind.

One year, a few of us heard the deep rhythm of drums somewhere out in the darkness and, that same night, we saw faces pressed up against the windows, strange and yet familiar dark eyes looking in on us. We felt as though we were in a circle of great power, one that had enclosed us in protection and in love. The outside world, the world of television and phones and cars and technology, had never felt so far away as it did that night. To belong again...

It can be a terrible, lonely thing to have wandered so far from our homes, from the spirits that we all once knew, the spirits of the Old World and of the Old Forest. This New World that we have come to has its own spirits, but we have not really gotten to know them, let alone form the sort of bonds we had with the Earth spirits back in Europe. Not like how our ancestors knew the land.

The people of the past spoke to the spirits of the land and the spirits spoke back in their own way. They needed to know the Earth intimately because the fertility of their fields and crops depended on it, and by extension their very lives. They did not just take and take, sure that it was their right to do so, uncaring of what might happen when the resources at hand would eventually run out. They knew they were a part of the cycle and that the future was dependant upon the past, as the peoples' good fortune and lives were intertwined with the good fortune and life of the land.

People in the Western World today have pretty much forgotten this lesson, as they have forgotten themselves. Mother Earth is mother to us all and She loves us, yes, ever and always, She loves us. And, thankfully, She has far more patience than most of us could ever hope to understand. But that does not mean that She will turn a blind eye forever to what the human race does to this planet, nor that She may not choose at some time to end what is and begin something new. After all, She has done it many times before. Nothing modern technology or science may do and nothing it knows, or thinks it knows, can stop Her in that eventuality. Hurricanes, tornados, earthquakes, and tidal waves are just some of Her more visible powers.

We are at Her mercy and, thankfully, She tends towards mercy. Even though, for a long time now, some religions have taught that the world and the things of the world are wicked and that nature is Herself evil. Just as they have taught that it is the *right* of humankind to have absolute dominion over the whole Earth and do what they like with it, even to the extent of destroying the environment and slaughtering entire species. Understandably, how may we connect and love the Earth and respect Her, so long as that belief holds sway over us.

A mother's patience is long, but a good mother does not protect her children from their own folly. If she did, then they would never learn and grow on their own. It is a fool's faith to deny and destroy what we all need to survive and to ignore how all of life is linked together on this planet. We need to stand up and be responsible, both for our own actions and for the world that we are passing down to our children. We need to learn to take the long view, maybe not as long a view as the Earth spirits and Mother Earth is capable of, but we must try our best all the same. For by coming to a proper respect for Her, we also begin to respect ourselves and the living creatures we share this world with.

Earth is the most silent and least understood of all the elements, yet we are drawn to understand it all the same, as best we can, for without that understanding and connection we have no future. It is a necessity for us to come to form those bonds once more so that when we walk upon the ground, when we thread the maze, travel the labyrinth to its very core, we begin to feel the beat of the world through own our flesh and know its rhythm in our bones.

We are not so different from those we share this world with, for we all share the same Mother. Wherever we go, She goes with us. Our physical forms are made of Her, flesh and bone we belong to the Earth and our history exists not just in books, in the written word, but is built into our very bodies, in the memories that lie hidden in our bodies. We all share these memories—the memory of where we all came from, the cave of the Mothers, where was worked the Mother's magick, the rituals passed down through the Priestesses of the land.

Far back in time, we lived as one with the Earth and learned to call the power of fire to our hand, and when storms came, when lightnings flashed and water poured down and the wind made the forests dance...we felt the energy of that pour itself into our bodies and wash us anew as it washed the land anew.

Some of these magicks still exist today, especially in the native religions who still understand the concept of belonging to same family as that of animals and fish and birds and even the plants. They remember that we are brothers and sisters, all of us children of the same Earth Mother. This has come down to us as the power of totem magick, of belonging to the clan of one creature or another and sharing in that magickal legacy.

Animal totems are another reminder of the time when we walked as one with the powers of storm and of bird and bEast and desired to know what they could teach us. Out of this desire, we became of the same family as they, blood of their Blood, clan of their clan. Their powers and talents became our own and have come down through our descendants, though—like Witch Blood—it has also grown thin through the years and difficult to awaken.

Still, the natural instincts have remained inside us, instincts and the ancient blood connection. When you reconnect to the Earth, you also relearn what it means to have shared blood with other living creatures. Whether that blood is that of a bird, such as a raven, or an animal, such as a cat. Spiders, stags, bears, snakes, flowers, owls, wolves, all of them had something to impart to our ancestors, just as they have much to show us today.

Connecting to the animal spirits, who are our kin, helps us to remember what it's like to live in close companionship to the Earth Mother. As with the spirits of each place, there is also a greater animal spirit for each kind of animal. This greater spirit embodies the attributes of that particular species and is, in a way, the living group consciousness which binds all of them together as one. In this way, you don't just connect to ravens or wolves or cats or owls, but to Raven, to Wolf, to Cat, or to Owl. You connect to that which all ravens or wolves take their form and essence from.

As a King is the living representation of his people and as the Gods and Goddesses represent different aspects or elements, so each animal spirit represents not just all the other animals they are kin to, but the powers and inherent characteristics of that animal. All larger spirits contain within them smaller spirits, and a group of smaller spirits can come together to create a larger conscious spirit. While the greatest spirit of them all—what the Lakota call *Wakan Tonka*, but who has had many names in many cultures—embodies all the spirits everywhere and is the Source of us all.

Depending then on your bloodline, you may have it within you to be a part of Raven or a part of Owl, whatever creature your ancestors formed a bond with. Since we have interbred so much over the generations though, you may have many different possibilities inside you. One may be stronger than another though, or one may be more needed in your life or in your community, and this is likely to be the one you will finally make contact with and awaken within you.

Akin to Earth spirits, you can't have a true bond with more than one at a time, though. If you are kin to Bear and have formed a link with Bear—having acknowledged Bear in your blood and awoken that particular talent and power—then you cannot go and form a link with another animal spirit at the same time, such as with Eagle or Wolf or Cat. Animal spirits can be as possessive as Earth spirits in that way. But then they each have a lot to teach us, more than one person can learn in a lifetime, and so pursuing a strong and deep relationship is to the benefit of us all.

One of the things that they can teach us is how to have silent non-verbal communion, a trait that they share with the spirits of the Earth. As well as how to trust in our deeper instincts, in the ways we can flow in tune with the land and with the energies within the land. Especially since it's reflective of the way that energies flow through our own bodies, as the greater always reflects the smaller and the smaller, the greater.

The Path of Service

How can Witches help and guide mankind if they do not shine?
If Witches are not beautiful or honorable or compassionate or believe in service to both
the Gods and the good of the land.
If they do not know how to love or how to laugh in pure joy?

One teaches by example, by being all that you wish others to aspire to.

One of the reasons why a Witch is here, is to teach. Not just to teach others to be Witches, though it's a necessary role to aid in raising the next generation to take the Craft into the future, but to help guide and teach of all humanity. Being a Witch means taking an intrinsic role in the human quest towards understanding itself, towards peace, love, creativity, and true power.

There are spirits all around us and some of those spirits are dedicated towards the same goal, towards guiding and teaching those of us here on the Earth who live in the physical world. These spirits can take on many forms, many aspects, but one thing remains true about them—all higher spirits are beautiful in their own way. They are generous, honest, kind and exactly what you need at this particular time in your life. This doesn't mean that they can't be stern when necessary, because though they are here to help and guide and protect, they are not here to solve all your problems for you. That would be a disservice in their part, the same as if they ended up making your issues worse.

Higher spirits, higher souls, are not petty or greedy or controlling and they are definitely not self-involved. Like Earth spirits, they take the longer view and look at what you most require in your life in order to be able to grow, both as a person and as a spirit. They are teachers in every aspect because they know that the greatest gift you can give to someone is the ability for them to discover and walk their own path, to fill themselves with their own light and life and power.

However, a gift like that can't just be handed over, all neatly wrapped and packaged. The most any teacher can do is try to impart to a student the tools that they need in order to go there themselves, in order to gain access to their own inmost divine gifts. And the best way a teacher has of doing that is to be an example. In short, you have to let your own higher spirit shine out through you so that you can teach others to do the same.

The soul of another is a trust and when you become their teacher a bond is formed between you. What is entrusted to you in this way you have to protect, even from your own worst whims and habits, your lacks and failings. You must act out of your better instincts and always strive to be more than yourself, to be your own *higher* self, if you are going to be another's guide. You must allow higher forces to work through you, whether that means otherworldly beings, elementals, or different Gods and Goddesses.

To teach others, you must be honest and wise and creative and strong as you can be. You must know when to speak and when to keep your silence. You must know what to strive for and keep that focus in the face of all the world if need be, so long as what you strive for is what the world requires best. You must allow the powers of creation to work through you. And you must be honest, both with others and with yourself, above all else.

Your own good word must always mean something. Your own good name must always mean something. For, without that you are holding fast to nothing and lies can become so much a part of you that you will no longer be able to tell the difference between them and the truth. You risk becoming a shadow of your own soul, rather than the light. Definitely, you will not be living the life that the Divine meant for you to live.

In order to rightly teach, you must be a righteous teacher. You must walk the correct path, the path that leads you to being a beacon of light in the dark—the same path that leads to your purest self, to who you really are, or, in other words, the path of the Quest. Because you cannot teach others to know what it is to be pure if you are not on the same road. The road which leads past mirrors and monsters, the challenges of the journey that are there in order to test you and so allow you to gain in power and understanding.

Part of this understanding means being able to tap into the flow of the Craft, into the powers of the Old Ways. For this reason, an Elder is someone who can guide and judge and give advice because they touch the heart of the Craft and know what is best for it. They have come to the point where they no longer seek gain for themselves and don't judge or rule just from their own life's experiences, but adjudge according to the long term good of the Craft.

Elders and teachers and guides are those Witches that the powers speak through, who have learned how to set aside ego so that the Craft may act through them as much as they act in the Craft. The Blood is a living thing and you need to learn how to touch the roots of it and find eternal renewal. Then you can rule not out of short term concerns such as hate or anger or fear or want, but out of the living essence of all of Witches past and future.

Elders can and must see the big picture and take the long road, without losing track of what it means to live in the sometimes painful now. They have to understand the nature of sacrifice, not the sacrifice of one's true self, but sacrifice in order to *attain* one's true self, one's proper place in the world. They must see what the world and what the Craft needs and set into motion what will fulfill that need. This embodies the strength of the Craft, as joy and pleasure provide the beauty—both of which are needed if you are to come to an understanding of love.

Plainly put, in joy and in love we may attain the realms of the Gods, but our bodies also need to be fed and clothed and made comfortable because otherwise their needs will distract us. More than that, through attending to physical needs, we can also feed the spiritual aspect of our selves. The two can become one and expand beyond the two halves of the whole. This is different from the path of the past two thousand years, where people have been taught to tear the two apart and focus only on the spiritual, ignoring and even denigrating the physical.

Witches never lost touch with the physical world, though. Indeed, we revel in it. Witches don't seek to "escape" from the Earth, for Witches were born to be guardians of this world. Witches are in their own way as tied to the land—or should be—as much as any other elemental being. Even though their origins are of the heavens, they are also born of the Earth, of the cave of the Earth Mother. It is from this place that Elders must learn to speak. Not with their own singular voice, but with the voices of Witches of old, the Witches of all time. With the voice of that which is Witch, as much as Bear speaks for all bears everywhere and Raven speaks for all ravens.

Elders need to be channels for powers that are necessary to the Earth, both powers that maintain order and powers that bring change. Elders need to be able to touch who they have been, calling upon the wisdom of past lives and of the spirit which stands central of all they were and will be. This gives them the ability to be able to see not just what the Earth needs, but what each individual student needs and what place they are meant to have in the Craft and in the world, what they are here to accomplish.

It's a fine balance, one where the Elder has to let the natural forces and the Gods work through them, while keeping in mind the best interests of the Craft, of the community, and of the student. After all, this is the next generation being raised, the next wave of healers and teachers, guardians and guides. Those who will, in turn, give birth to their own teachers in due time, as the cycle of life, death, and rebirth continues. Above all, Elders must be able to see the journey. Maybe not in specific detail all the time, but that each life is a movement in a greater symphony, one with both beautifully tragic notes and terribly joyful ones.

But Witches look not just to the sky and to the Earth, but to the moon and to the sun. The sun gives both light and love, while the moon gives shadow and peace. To stand in the middle of the moon is to know the love of the sun, and yet to have the peace of the world's blessings. To stand in the middle of the sun is to know the shadow you yourself cast into the world and to know your own light. In this way, we are all made of light and shadow, love and peace. Not warring factions, but a dynamic whole.

Everyone needs to find their own way to balance, to the core of what is right for them. In this way, none of us can seek to learn anothers' lesson, nor hand over the answers. If someone is not ready to hear or to understand those answers, it will mean nothing to them. Both are a disservice to the student. Instead, we all need to learn our own lessons and shine out as a beacon to show that it can be done.

This is a part of the dawning Age, to understood the light and comprehend the dark. To see each aspect within ourselves and know the peace and love that lies at the core of them, that lies where two meet and become one. The problem is that we have become so inured to struggle that even this sort of seeking is presented as a course of struggle and pain, not realizing there is also a road of joy and pleasure that can be taken. As well as a middle road which embraces them both.

The Gods do not choose which road we shall take. It is up to us to decide. In the Piscean Age, people were told they could pick only one road of two—the path of light which led to God or the path of darkness which led to the Devil. In the Aquarian Age, these roads will be braided back together again and Witches have to be the vanguard of the new path which shall emerge, the one of light and darkness intertwined in dynamic interplay and balance.

This is the middle road which acknowledges the deep connection between the physical and the metaphysical realms. It is the Faery road which leads over the rolling hills to the land of our ancestors and our descendants. The path of the moon and the sun, of light and love and shadow, and of the stars tumbled down to Earth to taste the pleasures of the flesh. This is the path of the God and of the Goddess, neither one supreme over the other, but finding themselves most alive, most adored in each other's eyes.

Light and love and shadow, all are aspects of the Divine fire which exists in each Witch and which must be loosed again upon the Earth in order to guide and to inspire. But to do this, you must know what love is, for love is both the key and the doorway. Love is what we explore in each and every ritual, for love is magick and magick is love. As to worship is also to love—to love the Gods—and so when we worship the Gods we love Them and we celebrate one of the greatest magicks of all.

Born of Beauty and of Strength

A hand's pass and mist rises,
Smoke and magick lie captive
Before the touch of silver to willing flesh,
And so the pattern is impressed
As would be writ upon living paper,
Upon the skin of dust and bone
Crushed and mingled into life
Or set as bread upon the plate;
A fEasting for all
Who would accept the price
And the tender touch
Of fate

What are rituals? Rituals are something that you do again and again, creating a pattern. A pattern engraves itself on the fabric of the universe as it engraves itself upon your heart. But where do rituals come from? All rituals have their source in the Gods and they are created out of need and out of necessity. Why do we do them? We do them for love. So rituals come to us from the Gods and out of need and we do them for love.

Rituals are, in their own way, masks because they are patterns and patterns groove things into the fabric of reality. The more a pattern is repeated, the stronger it becomes and the more power it takes onto itself. This pattern can then, eventually, become conscious in its own right, with the pattern as its living visible mask, as the Gods as living visible masks for greater powers.

In rituals, we tend to use symbols more than words because symbols can often touch us deeper. A lit candle can be a doorway, a gate to other realms. Salt and water to serve as symbols of purification, while our ahtames focus our personal will and power and energy. Even the circle itself is a symbol of the boundary between this world and the Otherworld, between what is known and what is as yet unknown.

When we use symbols in our rites, when we invoke and raise powers through our rituals, they take on form in order to enter our reality. In the same way, we are all ourselves symbols and masks through which the Unseen powers manifest. Every time a circle is called into being it forms a beacon in the outer darkness, a beacon which draws conscious powers to it; so you must be careful what you send out because what will respond shall be similar in nature. Like attracts like, so that if the Witches in a group are always at odds with each other or there are deep-seated fears and angers and resentments in the coven psyche, then the powers that will be drawn to the group may end up being angry or fearful or resentful ones.

It's an oversimplification of sorts, for individuals and covens are much more complex than that, but better to emphasize virtues rather than vices. If each Witch is honest and true to their self, then how much more honest and true will their coven be, the coven that they form from their combined hearts and dreams and voices. A coven becomes the embodiment, the consciousness, of all those who have pledged themselves to it. Together, they create a greater whole, a spirit song which can reach out across the void and take them to the far places, to where they need to go in order to bring back the gifts of the new Age.

Dark tides rise and fall, leaving behind the secrets of the sea. The sea keeps many secrets, the same as the Earth. But then they are both old, the sea Mother and the Earth Mother; They were there in the beginning, when the Lord of Fire also ruled. They have been cruel and kind in turn and yet their natures remain beyond our full comprehension for They think and feel in currents, deep and wide, one leading to another. As one Age leads to another, beginning in the deep places of the Earth and in the secret depths of the Water, leaving Witch and Faery to mold what comes from Fire and Air.

The Ages are markers of eternity and like every living thing, they rise to their heights only to falter and fall. They are born, as we are born, to eventually and inevitably die. Accordingly, there is also a spirit of each Age, a grand consciousness that grows to understanding of itself, as we who live each Age grow to an understanding of it. This is the "King" of the Age—the embodiment of all that Age is, was, and can be, its greatest glory and its greatest hope.

The elements of Fire, Earth, Water and Air form the foundation which must be built in order to raise the temple of each Age, with the heart as both the crown and the center. All journeys must, by nature, start with the heart for the heart is the door of understanding and to knowing your purest self. It leads to both to an outer world and an inner one, to the Divine flame which crowns the head and makes you a Shining One.

A King is a Shining One for a King becomes his heart. He speaks for the heart as he speaks for the world, standing in the center of the crossroads with the crown upon his head, a cup in one hand and a rod in the other. A King represents us all, because at that moment he *is* us all. He breathes when we breathe and his blood flows through us as ours flows through him. In this way, Kings are always of the North Quarter because they embody what it is to be *Being*.

The symbol of the crowned heart is one of the symbols of kingship. For a King is not made, but born by coming into the world with his heart intact. His only sin is to ever forget that, for only when he forgets who he is and that which he represents, is that connection lost. Each Age has its Quest as each Age has its King, the one who hasn't forgotten the secret of the Grail, the secret of his true nature. The aspect that each Quest takes depends upon the symbolism of the Age and what we need to learn as a species as we pass through the Ages one after the other.

A King does not need the Quest to know who he is, to find the source of his power, unless he makes the mistake of forgetting. But we do. We each need to make that journey in every lifetime so that we can become the Kings of our own lives, the Being of our own lives. So the Grail is different for everyone as it is different for each Age. But yet there are certain aspects of the Quest which remain consistent.

There is always the journey itself, during which you or the Age may acquire certain helpers along the path. For the dawning of each Age, these helpers have been called many things down through the centuries, but one word for them is an Avatar. They tend to be guides, healers, and teachers and they bring the form of light most needed to illuminate that particular Age. In some respects, they embody the virtues of their Age.

In each Witch's own personal journey, you can also acquire the aid of various helpers, Avatars to your own soul which can take the form of guides, healers, and teachers. Sometimes they may be actual physical people you come into contact with, friends or counselors or teachers or family members. At other times, they may not physically exist in this world at all, but be spirit guides who you can connect to and whose form will depend upon what you need and will respond to most in your life.

Like any true Avatar, these guides—whether they are here in the flesh or not—must be helpful and not harmful, though they will not, and nor should they, solve all your problems for you. Overcoming problems and facing issues are an intrinsic part of your journey, part of the tests you need to pass along the way. No one learns anything by having someone else handle their issues for them. Helping others is a good thing, but helping them to avoid their problems is not.

In this way, true spirit guides do not spend their time interacting with you in order to help you run away from your issues and, most definitely, they shouldn't make them worse. If they do, then they are not true spirit guides, but may indeed be inappropriate spirits who have been drawn to aspects of your anger, fears, and doubts which you have knowingly or unknowingly broadcast into the world. They may even be one of your own monsters masquerading as a guardian or helpful spirit.

A particular name for one of these monsters is the Guardian at the Gate, a monster who takes on the shape of your own worst doubts and fear and shame. You not only have to fight this monster, but you have to accept that whatever dark force the monster conceals is actually a part of you. You have to come to the realization that you created this monster yourself and that it takes not just its form from you, but its very life and power.

That does not mean that the secret that the Guardian at the Gate hides, the power that energizes it, is some great and evil force, some bad thing that is really a part of you. The energy itself is not a bad thing, it is just that the form it has taken for the time being is based on fear or doubt or shame or guilt or, worst of all, hatred. In order to truly defeat the monster you have to take back your power, transmuting it into a creative force that is to your own benefit and to the benefit of others.

This monster can take on many shapes—fear of quitting your job even when you hate it, fear of leaving someone you no longer love because you don't want to be alone, fear of going somewhere you've never been. It can be doubt of your own self-worth, doubt that you will ever find anyone to love and who will love you, or doubt that you can be successful. It can take the form of shame over who you are, who you want to be, or who you may have once been. There are many monsters and we often have more than one lurking about, which can entail having to face many personal tests.

But every time you face that test and face down that monster, you take back part of your own energy. Not only does this make you stronger, but it makes you able to see your own self better and you come closer to understanding why you are here and what wonderful things you are capable of. It won't completely smooth over the bumps in the road, but it will make you better able to withstand and overcome those bumps with greater confidence and strength. Your energy will, once more, be your own and not be going to feed your fears and insecurities.

In the Quest of the Age, the journey and the tests undertaken are a group effort, though often the vast majority of people do not really consciously know they are on a Quest. Those who willingly and knowingly take up the Quest of the Age are the vanguard of the future. They lead the way, lighting torches along the path so that those who come after can follow. They, too, may not entirely know where the Quest is taking them and the exact form of the Grail of the Age, but they have chosen to take up the challenge all the same.

This Quest takes hundreds of years to realize, but everyone can do their part, even if you are not in the vanguard. Taking up your own personal Quest and defeating your own personal monsters can only be an aid to all. You cannot be a light, nor light the path for others, if you have been consumed by darkness and allowed the monsters to take over your life. It takes a tremendous amount of energy away from you, energy that could be put to a better, more productive use.

When you take back your rightful power and energy it can feed you instead of your monsters, propelling your life into a lightness and vitality of body and spirit. Which is not to say that you should just go ahead and do whatever you feel because "it's all good," because what you do has to be in accord with your true self, which must be in accord with the will of the universe. Which means having to clarify your life so that you can know not only what that will is, but where your own will stands.

Not that everyone doesn't have doubts and fears, and they are not likely to just go away at the snap of your fingers. There are always more monsters out there. And not to say that, over time, it will become easy to face them—if it was it wouldn't be much of a test—but you will be able to face them with a greater sense of confidence and knowing that overcoming them will only help you in the long run. As it will help those around you.

But the Quest can be glorious as much as painful. It can be marked with joyful times as much as difficult ones. It takes the conscious choice, the willing heart, the courage to go forward, the ability to forgive, and love, most of all, love in order to face those monsters and succeed. If you fill yourself up with these things, then you will not only light the path for yourself, but leave a light behind for those who will come after. You will be a guide and a healer and a teacher by your own example of beauty and of strength.

The nature of the universe is both one of order and of chaos, not in conflict with each other but in dynamic balance. Ritual is a way to handle these powers by using a mask, symbol, or metaphor, because these powers are not otherwise available to us in their pure form. They are just too strong for our physical bodies to long withstand, so we have to create masks for them, windows and doors for them to filter into our world through a name, a shape, an image, or through an act of ritual.

All great powers form consciousnesses, and any consciousness can be given a name and through the power of that name enter into our reality and become "real." But it's like naming the tip of an iceberg—you can see it and touch it and know it, but yet the greatest part remains invisible and unknowable, even though that is the most dangerous and most powerful part of all. That's because the name of a great power is only the smallest piece of it, the piece that has extended itself into this world.

In this way, great powers are like spectrums which range from light which is visible to us to that which is not. It is all part of the same thing, but we can only see a portion of it. We can only know the part that has been funneled into our world through its living mask.

But what are the great powers?

Well, love is one of them, and who may truly think to name or define love? Though thousands have tried down through the ages, who has ever really fixed the least of it into place? Love is more than just a feeling, more than a concept, more than the physical or emotional expression of it. For love is the power that permeates the universe and works what might be called magick or miracles. To walk in love is to exist in an altered state, one where you are absolutely aware and at peace with both yourself and everything else.

When you walk in tune with your soul, which walks in tune with your spirit, which walks in tune with the Source, then you walk the path of love. Not denying the pain and sorrow of the world, anymore than the joys or pleasures, but transcending them all by being in the center. A center where you are moved by everything and nothing, seeing everything exactly for what it is and yet, standing removed from it at the same exact time.

Great powers take unto themselves masks of consciousness…and why not? The more complex an organism, the more likely it will achieve such a state and learn to think and feel for itself. If this is true for physical living beings, then why not for that which is living, but non physical such as various spirits and Gods and rituals and elemental beings.

This world is not the only one. What we see is not all there is. In order to truly see the universe, you have to learn the trick of seeing beyond what the five senses tell you it is. Science can only get you so far. Religion can only get you so far. At some point, you must leap beyond both and into the greater world that lies beyond the structure we attempt to impose upon it. You must stand in the hall of the Gods and see the masks of the powers staring down at you, and then to risk all, dare all, to see past even that.

It is a matter of choice and always is. It is a matter of knowledge and of faith, of trust and of risk. If you believe in hate and anger and emptiness then your world becomes hate and anger and emptiness. Your world becomes the wasteland. The wasteland is the loss of faith in love, in hope and in self. It is a loss of the light of love, which is the true face of the

Source. To best express your own light you must learn to express love…to live and walk and be with love. So the Quest is as much within as without, for to express love you must first seek it within and then make of yourself a pure and shining gate for that same light and love.

To do this you must be made pure, so what is not of your own true self must be left behind. It must be purged and stripped away, sloughed off, so that all that remains is what is proper for you. Like wheat being separated from the chaff, you have to endure the process of losing what is not really you to begin with but what you may feel desperate to keep and cling to all the same.

Not that this Quest isn't a choice, because we are always given a choice. Though change is inevitable, how we choose to react to that change is always in our own hands. It is up to us to decide if we will work with the onrushing tide or whether we will make the attempt to swim against it. It is up to us to decide whether or not to deny or to accept gladly the workings of fate, the shining web of the stars and the glimmering candles which light the stage upon which we perform God's play. For choice came with the gift of Fire.

The Quest takes us to the farthest boundaries that can be imagined and farther still. It takes us both within and without, to the cave of the beginnings and beyond the boundaries of all that is known. So while the Lady of the Quest holds out the cup of the Quest to each of us, She also holds out a mirror, for to drink from the cup is to drink from the well of self and to see who we really are.

We must all cross the river, go past the boundaries and venture into the great beyond. We must all make the leap of faith and look into the mirror. We must all drink from the cup, the cup with is also the Lady's well, the well of blessings which is fed from the deepest rivers of the Earth. The well wherein you can see the sparkle of the farthest stars, dreams and visions all. The well and cup and mirror of the Quest and of pure love.

A love which does not own. A love which has nothing to do with false pride or with despair or ego. A love which knows all things come and go as they must, as they will, and the only good fool is the one who believes and trusts in that and in himself, and so becomes King for the day. For the King and the Fool are both sides of the same coin, one the face of knowing and one the face of faith.

The Lady of the Well, the Lady of the Quest, is the White Lady. Gwenhyvar is one of Her names and She is the guide, beckoning with Her own ethereal beauty to call us to exceed our own expectations. You can find Her in the Arthurian legends, though what She seems there has as much to say about Christian virtues and legends as it does about the Pagan ones which long preceded them. In Christian parlance, Guenivere is soft and gentle and pure—and her fall from grace with Lancelot resulted in Arthur's loss of knowledge of his own Kingship and created the wasteland.

This is a rather simplistic retelling of an old truth. Guenivere is soft and gentle and pure as a teacher, but as she is also a mirror, she reflects our own fears and desires. She is the whiteness, the brightness, but she is also the dark, because love is never just one-sided. Love is both beautiful and terrible, and so must the Queen of Love be, the Queen of the Quest for Love. She would be soft for us, tender for us, but the truths in Her mirror are not soft, they are not tender, and they can burn equally well.

Still, what you find at the end of the Quest is not something that is soft and gentle, for it is beyond beauty as we know it here. It is light that is dark and dark that is light. It is something so lovely that it hurts to even behold it. So, in order to bring it back with us, to return with any part of what we find, we can only return with what can fit behind the mask we make for it.

Gifts and Revelations

Turn and bind the ribbons bright
Strike into the cauldron's might
Work to weave the spell aright
From maypole to the tomb
Dance to bring the light within
Dance to know the darker ring
Sons and daughters of the line
Of bell and book and broom

A gift makes a connection; it binds the giver to the receiver and should not be given lightly, nor lightly received. It is an exchange of the heart, which makes the most powerful part of a gift not so much the actual physical object or service given, but the feeling behind it, the connection. A connection which has an effect on both the giver and the receiver.

Gift giving is a form of reciprocity, a way of keeping the bounty of the universe vital and flowing. Bounty is energy in essence, even if sometimes that energy is manifested in physical objects. To give a gift is to give of your own energy—even more so if you have, in fact, made the gift—and so to share something of who you are with another. You can more clearly see that in the past, when people tended to make gifts for each other, rather than go out and buy them at a store. They put their energies into what they made, even if they didn't deliberately put a magickal wish into them.

The bountiful spirit of Yule, a spirit and God who has come to be known in many countries as Santa Claus, Saint Nicholas, among other names, is a personification of that giving energy. Santa Claus does not give out of any expectation of return; he simply gives because it is in his nature to give. It's part of who he is. He provides the example that it is actually in *all* of

276

our natures to be able to give of our selves, for by being your best self you provide a gift to the world.

When you go on the Quest, you become capable of bringing more and more of that energy into being. As you pass the tests on the journey and gain each treasure, one more facet of the jewel of your soul is polished and the whole shines all the more brightly for it. Until what you bring into being is not just your own singular self, but your past lives and your future and all the aspects of the Higher Spirit to which you belong, all the facets scattered across space and time.

You go on the Quest to find those other facets, just as you go on the Quest to bring back gifts meant for your loved ones, your family, coven, and community. Gifts which can take the form of new and wonderful ideas and concepts, as yet unknown and unrealized. Including revelations from the eternal possibility of the Divine, for whatever can be dreamt of or imagined is one step closer to being realized in the world of flesh and form.

These things happen all the time. These things happen all around us. Sometimes, it's just time for something to come into being and suddenly people from all over will get a similar idea, a similar thought, as if the idea was reaching out to anyone who could hear it, who might be open to receive it. This happens to writers all the time and to those in the movie and television industry—they start working on a project only to discover later that another person began working on an eerily similar project at almost exactly the same time. It's not that anyone "stole" the idea from someone else, as neither knew the other, but more like they had both tuned into the same "broadcast," into an idea whose time had simply come.

These expressions are shaded by the artist who is trying to bring it into being, of course. It must come through their skills and talents and experiences, so no two efforts will be identical even if the core idea was the same. Still, you can often see the core, the kernel, the seed of the idea no matter what trappings it is hiding within, what mask it now wears. As if each was creating a shadow in order to try to catch a glimpse of the light behind it, a beautiful light that could not fully appear in our world, due to the constraints of matter. Which leaves the only way to "see" by working to fashion a mask for it, a shadow, the visible tip of a great invisible iceberg.

If the spirit world, the Otherworld, is the light, then this world is the shadow. The two are intimately connected across the boundary that many have come to call the Veil, and both have a natural, mutual, and profound effect upon each other. When you gain the Second Sight, you find the ability to see with the heart, to see through the boundary, beyond the Veil. This is a necessary talent if you want to travel to the Otherworld and to other worlds, in general. How can you go there unless you can see? How can you return again unless you can see?

To go, to travel, to see past the mask, to play the Game, to take the tests, and to reclaim some missing part of the universe, some precious gift and jewel meant for all of humanity...it's not easy, but yet it's not impossible either, especially since the universe itself desires us to succeed. Help and aid is always there to be called upon, companions "for the road," as it were. If you act in good faith, in honesty, with honor and truth in your heart, then good and honorable and true company will always come to you.

For in the spirit world—and in this world, for that matter—those that you draw to you always come for a reason and at the behest of the energies that you send out. Like attracts like, and so the necessity of truly coming to know yourself and of finding your balance, of having a strong and flexible foundation. Because if you wish to bridge worlds, you will need both strength and the ability to bend, as well as a good and true intent.

Humility comes into play, as well, real humility, because the gifts that we seek, the gifts that we bring back, are not meant for us. We will benefit from them, no doubt, but that can't be why you go after them in the first place. You can't undertake the journey solely for yourself anymore than the focus can be on what you might get in return.

You have to *give* without any thought of *getting* or it's not really a gift at all. Even worse is the thought of keeping some sort of tally of what is owed for what you have done, for what you have risked, for what you have sacrificed—which makes what you have given neither a gift nor a sacrifice. You must do it simply because you desire to do it, because you have found it in your nature to give, because it has become part of your bliss to do so. And it must always stem from love.

The impetus must be love and the form must be love, especially since a gift is a kind of magickal act. It's an energy that binds things together, that creates a living web of connection. You can see this energy in the way that the gifts of the Gods to humankind formed an accord and bound the fates of the two together. As well as in the way we give to the Gods and the Gods give to us, forging a relationship of mutual love, support, and need.

Fascination is often the first way this kind of love makes itself known, for fascination fixes the attentions and opens the door of the heart, without which nothing can really be given or received. A locked heart can do neither and risks becoming like stagnant water or stony land, where nothing good can grow. In order to be creative and fertile and loving, one must have a willing heart, because what comes into existence in the cold and in the dark are deceptive things, empty creatures which would suck the light and warmth from the world if they could. Hollow inside instead of filled with light and life, the fire which was the first, best gift of the Gods.

Not that it is easy to give without expectation, especially when we are raised with a fear of lack, that there just isn't enough good things to go around. It seems natural and smart then to become stingy, to hoard, to hold things close, rather than to let the free flow of energy surge through us and through our lives. But letting powers and energies work through us is part of what being a Witch is all about and having an open heart is the main key to working the greater magicks, to regaining what has been lost over the centuries, including who and what we are as Witches.

Midnight, the Witching Hour, has come at last and the Witches stand in a circle, holding hands around a central spark. They stand ready to call upon the old powers and to dance in the old ways. To dance in the flesh and to dance in spirit, to Dance the Blood and know who they once were, who they are, and who they can be. As at the dawn of this next great Age, we stand ready to be reborn, to come again into what has long been thought lost. We stand ready to pick up the pieces and form a bridge, a foundation, a great tower reaching upwards to the heavens.

There is a Witch way and a Witch culture and a Witch history that the modern world either has come to out-and-out deny or to claim that it is nothing much more than wish fulfillment, the twisted remnants of myth and superstition. They point fingers and say our ancestors were simple and uneducated and that times are so much better now, that we know so much more today. But do we? A Witch knows that what the modern world believes it knows is just different from that of the past, not necessarily better. That, in fact, the world of the ancients, of mingled wonder and terror, magick and transformation is still here, all around us, buried deep inside us, if only we have eyes to see it.

Yes, some would call them fairytales, but what are fairytales except the lingering remnants of ancient stories of Gods and spirits and magick and dreams. Of men and Witches and the powers that came long before the cross, the powers of sea and of forest, of sky and earth and stream. Perhaps, the idea of faeries being small happened in part because man could no longer imagine—or no longer wished to believe—that there were greater things out there than himself. That there were, and still remain, things that are beyond thought, beyond comprehension, beyond reason and logic. That humans are not necessarily the top of the spiritual food chain.

If we wish to reclaim the powers of the past, to see as our ancestors saw, we have to change how we think and how we look at things. It's a gift that the past has to give us, as well as all those Witches who came before us and gave of the Blood so that we could be reborn to them. Still, it's never easy to change, especially knowing you have to start inside, start with yourself. But if belief is faith and faith is fate, then we create our own fates, even in the face of destiny.

Destiny is what is written in the stars, into the very fabric of the universe, what the universe wills, but fate...fate can change. Fate can change if you believe long and hard enough to change it. But you must *really* believe, perfectly and absolutely, for only then will your faith bring a new world into being, the new world you have made the choice to live in. It can't just be a surface belief, but one that reaches all the way through you, all the way to your core foundation. This intensity of belief is one of the gifts of the Old Ones.

The journey of learning how to internalize the powers of the Four Quarters—of making them your foundation—gains for you the gifts necessary to succeed. For when someone is said to be gifted, it means that they have talents and abilities that aren't considered "normal" or "average." All it really means, though, is that they have become open to the potentials they were born with, that they have tuned into the creative energy that is being freely broadcast throughout the universe and have found a way to channel it.

Everyone has a gift. Everyone has a talent. Everyone has something special they can offer the world. Knowing is one of these gifts, as well as Doing and Daring and Being. They are the gifts offered to us by the Quarters and if you accept them they can form the basis for building something even greater and for further journeys, for bringing other sorts of gifts into being. Gifts of new ideas, beautiful stories, revelations, wonders, inventions, concepts not yet conceived of, lives never before lived, everything from a brand new breed of rose to a form of dance that no one has done before. Even a character in a movie unlike any other, one that influences people's lives and can even come to change the world.

Because gifts stem from Daring, from emotion and inspiration, it's quite natural for them to catch on and inspire others to dare, to feel and to become further sources of inspiration. For what comes from inspiration quite naturally inspires. The connection surges to life, like a stone cast into a still pond throws out ripples, or maybe the better metaphor would be rain falling into still water, where each droplet causes ripples and all the ripples meet and have an effect on each other.

Whatever can be dreamt of can be brought into reality, but dreams come first and they have to be born. You bring back a dream, you give it life and energy, and people begin to notice it, to tap into it. One dream spins off more dreams. These dreams take on a life, a consciousness of their very own. They find a way into physical reality, where their effect grows and the world begins to change. All from a dream. All from a gift. All from what is revelation—the revealing of something from beyond what is known, from the realm of Gods and dreams and spirits and Other.

Midnight is the hour when Witches wake the dream, when we stand at the center of the Wheel, the center of the crossroads, knowing it's a gateway to many realms, including the door of rebirth. As it's a gateway for ideas to enter into our reality, a gateway formed by the minds, hearts, and bodies of the Witches themselves, by the circle between the worlds.

As we in the circle raise our voices together, we build a wordless sound that twists and twines upward even as it reaches out into the beyond, a song that raises a beacon in the greater darkness. As the Witches create a great fire with the sparks within themselves, phoenix-fire, so hot that it is pure white at the core, it rushes outwards at the same time as it rushes inwards, revealing the landscape of promise and potential, of dream and desire. It reveals hills and deep valleys and secluded mountains, fallen-down castles and great earthen mounds. A forest with trees so huge you could hold a circle within their hollow trunks. Thickets where foxes flirt with great cats and where rabbits pause, their eyes like black buttons. And, where a white stag suddenly appears in the gloom, his horns upraised to hold a faintly glowing golden crown, a ruby at its heart.

Revealing a fire built of bones. A cave of bear skulls where women gather, their skin covered with clay and with dirt. Where a blue-skinned hag lifts gnarled hands to call the winters' storm, with frost-driven wolves by her side. Where a man dances in the meadow, with a mask of horn and paint, dancing to the pulse of a drum, that only he could hear. The winds rising, shadows crossing before the moon to the sound of distant hounds, the hunt just begun...

All this and more is there, most of which has been forgotten, but which can return again. It can be reclaimed from the dark, by the power of gifts and revelations. By waking again to what we once were, to what the deepest part of us never forgot, nor ever could. For the Blood is a gift as much as it also renders us capable of going to where we need to go in order to bring back gifts.

Some insist that the Witches of today have no real history. But we do. They make that mistaken claim or insistence in part, perhaps, because our true history is not written in books, but exists directly in the Blood. It's a living history, and one that can always be reclaimed and renewed because it *is* a living history. For those who die, die but to be born again, and those who are called to be Witches at this time are but the same Witches we knew in the distant past, even if some of them have yet to remember that. There's no broken line here, no shattered chain...for we are as we will be, as we once were, as we will be again.

The lives and spirit of a Witch form a circle, not a line. A circle with a life of its own, with a consciousness, a purpose, and a path. For it's a living spirit, one that all Witches are an intimate part of, as we are all part of the same fire as that of the stars. The fire, which was also a gift.

To Be Free

We are the dancers in the dark
Those who whisper spells
Along the tattered rim of reality
Flashing eyes and drifting hair
Pale feet
Naked upon the earth
Our hearts lie open and glittering
Like a thousand jewels
Upon the air
Upon the sky
As much a part of the great
Spell of spells
As any other weaver of dreams

Knowing is one of the elements of the East, the metaphysical aspect of Air, as Doing is the metaphysical aspect of Fire. When the spirit of a Witch is not invested in flesh they become of the Air, as when they take on physical form they are a being of Fire. But Air, of course, remains a part of them, Air which is breath, which is spirit. Which makes the inherent sort of Knowing which is the gift of the Eastern Quarter something that a Witch is born with.

Knowing is part of the heritage of the Old Ones, but it's not the kind of knowing that comes out of books. No, this kind of knowing is complete and instantaneous, complex and simple at the same time. It's not the kind of knowing of two plus two equals four or of building a case or an argument for something. It just *is*...suddenly and powerfully you just *know*. You know as though a door had suddenly opened itself up inside you. You know as though an intense light had just appeared, revealing what you couldn't see until that moment.

Once Priestesses breathed in sacred smoke and saw to the reality of the world beyond time and form. The words that they spoke came from that place of seeing were *sooth*, rather than *truth*. Sooth actually means divine reality, that which *is*, rather than truth which is made by humankind, truth which can change. One is a thing of the Gods and one a thing of man. The problem is that, over time, the meanings of the word sooth and of the word truth have been sWitched around, so that people tend to see truth as being that which is absolute. While sooth has been reduced to little more than illusion or fantasy, so much so that "soothsayers" tend to be considered charlatans and liars.

But soothsayers are the ones really telling it like it is. They have caught a glimpse of the real world behind the mask and are making the attempt to pass that knowledge along. Knowledge that they, themselves, might not comprehend later—or even consciously remember—and knowledge that doesn't always make sense to our more linear and rational minds. Which is why it's said that oracles often spoke in riddles, or in what seemed like riddles, because what they had to impart can be hard to express in any other way.

The Knowing of the East is a sort of seeing which encompasses all things. It's using a sense that is beyond the five physical senses. It's seeing the world from an altered state, a perceptual shift that allows us to take note of connections we otherwise are fairly oblivious to, connections that transcend both time and place. In the past, this altered state once was called by some "grace."

When you see through the eyes of grace, the world changes and yet is doesn't change at the same time; you simply have become one and at peace with it, as you have become one and at peace with your self, your soul, your eternal spark. People are not primarily what we see with our eyes; they are what we see and know with our heart. We see what binds us together as one, both as spirits and in the flesh. It shows us that we only imagine we are all alone and it's that imagining which makes us feel loss, loneliness, separation from self, others, and from the Divine.

The first Witch's circle was already a reflection. Like the sky mirrored in a beautiful and perfect lake, it exists in two worlds at once—the world above and the world below—and so all worlds lie transfixed between the two, endless and eternal. The first Witch's circle was made of stars and formed a crown of light, but because it's a reflection, a shadow as much as the light, there is something else which came before it. That something else is the pre-curser to all Witch's circles and so gave them their proper form, the mold from which they are cast.

It's the true Witch's circle, the one that takes place upon the Witch's Mountain, that transpires at Benevento, Blockula, Venusburg. For everytime a Witch draws a circle here on the Earth, it's matched by one in the heavens, a circle created by the spirits of the Air, the spirits of the dead, the spirits of the Otherworld. Each circle then is two-fold, shadow and light, here and there, ancient and new. All that we believe a Witches' circle should be, what it is meant to be, is realized where worlds meet.

The first pattern is the one of Knowing. When the circles that Witches create comes into alignment with that first circle, then those within the circle can know as they all knew when they were still spirits of Air. Then they can see and know the world behind the mask and more effectively change things, because of being closer to the powers and energies that imbue the physical world with life and power. As the Otherworldly circle is about Knowing, so the Witches' circle in this world is about Doing. When Knowing and Doing are linked, the result is enlightenment among other things, being consumed by the fire of knowledge.

One possible metaphor for the universe both Seen and Unseen is that of a spinning top. As it turns, so all aspects of light and dark, of life and of death, pass from one side to the other. We who live and die and live again—we of the East and of the South—exist upon the part of the top which spins. While the pole which causes the spinning is the place of Daring, the power of the West. At the center then, where the top spins so very fast that is has, in fact, ceased to spin, is the North. The North, which is the pivot point of the heavens, the pole star and the source of paradox.

In this way, the North is the center, as the West is the pole—the pillar down which the Unseen energies come into the world, the pillar which is also rainbow and a snake—and East and South are life and death in constant flux and dynamic balance. When you spin a top, you are seeing the Four Quarters in interaction, as well as time and eternity. It is a symbol of how the foundational powers work with each other, a metaphor for how the universe functions.

In much the same way, the symbol of the traditional pointed Witch's hat is not simply some silly artifact of a folk tale, for it represents the power of the Witch, of how the Witch's circle can create energies that rise up in a spiral towards the sky. This spiral eventually comes to a point and this point is then met by the powers that have spiraled downwards to meet it. It's for this reason that churches have towers, especially pointed towers—to try and draw down to the Earth the power of the skies, the power of the heavens. A lightning rod, if you will, for the bolt of the Gods.

So, too, an equal-armed cross is an old symbol, much older than the Christian usage of it, especially an equal-armed cross encompassed by a circle. Here you see the four powers of Earth, Air, Fire, and Water, plus the rim which brings them together to form a whole. Though, of course, the four lines that spring outward from the central point can also be seen as simply two lines, these two lines dividing the circle in equal halves. In this way, the lines represent life and death, light and dark, the crossroads where Witches meet and dance. Though to truly understand this particular symbol, you have to learn to see it in something other than a mere two-dimensional way, the same as with the figure eight which is a symbol of eternity on one hand and a symbol of life and death, this world and the Otherworld, at the same time.

A five-pointed star is also a symbol of long association with Witches, but a star can also properly be called a circle for it touches upon all the elements required, going round and back again. For example, if you begin in the North, go to the East, South, West, and return once more to the North, having touched five points in the process of drawing the circle, you have also completed a star. In this way, a circle is a star and a five-pointed star is a circle and so recalls to us the origin of the *Sorgitza*, and the history and source of their power.

In truth, there is never one thing without there being another. No symbol means just one thing, for it's in the nature of symbols to form connections. Just as no circle is ever drawn without there being a ripple, ripples through time and ripples through space, plus a connection back to the very first circle which gave rise to all the others throughout history. A circle that has as its center the same fire which is a spark of the Source, which is also the spinning/unspinning central pillar, as well as being the well of memory. In this fashion, a Witch's circle is a wheel and a crown and a star and a flame and a spiral and, that old standby, a conical hat pointed directly at the heavens, all at the same time and all of them equally real.

When you know as the Witches of old knew, when you see as they saw, then you will see in metaphor, in poetry, in riddle, in story, in legend and it will all make sense to you. Even if that sense is difficult, if not impossible most of the time, to express through our modern languages and sensibilities. To be able to talk about these kinds of visions, we have to speak in a language that can handle them, one that can express multiple meanings at the same time and is not essentially linear in nature. A language which has the ability to connect the name of a thing to the thing itself.

Not surprisingly, it's from this sort of connection came the idea that to name a thing was to call it into existence. Words do have that power, but only words that *know*, or that inspire one to *know* as you use them. The old Witch language has that power if you learn how to connect yourself to it. But, as this language has all but been forgotten, so the power of this kind of knowing has pretty much been lost, as well. It can be regained, however, by the stirring to life of the Blood, which is what the Old Ones, the ancient Witches, and the Old Gods desire for us to do.

Sons and daughters of the first circle, they know us when we build our circles upon the Earth and reflect the patterns of the night sky. They see our rising flame, hear our song, and know it for one of their own. As they know us for their own. It is their desperate wish to call us home again and to have us remember not just who we are and why we are here, but and all the joy and pleasure that can mean. Much has been lost, but with their encouragement and help it can be found again.

We can regain the ability to know and see and feel not just them, but each other, the Gods, and all there is. To find the freedom granted by the power of choice, the power of Fire inside each of us, and to link that Fire with the Knowing of the spirit, which is also inside us. Because when you Know and you Do, you bring a great light into the world, the light of divine illumination, that which makes us all as Shining Ones.

To know who you are and why you are here and to joyfully act out of that knowledge is to bridge the veil between this world and the Otherworld, to bring them together in communion and accord. It is real freedom, the freedom to be your own bliss, what the Divine has called you here to be. Only then, will you feel as you felt as a child, when all the wonders and possibilities of this world remained before you. When there were no closed doors, no regrets, no fear and no doubt inside your heart. For to know who you are is to be free to be who you are, as to know both beauty and strength inside you is to know love.

The Art

Time the perfect measure breaks
The heart it cannot fill
Have you the soul
Have you the strength
To bear the turning mill
Blood and bone to grind between
The heavy stones of old
Dust and wine
In taste sublime
Made a wheaten cake of gold.

Ariadne is the Muse, most beautiful, desirable, and terrible. She is the Goddess of inspiration, the wild flow of creativity that artists seek and yearn to tap into when creating and performing their best work, the kind that affects the world around them. When you touch Her, you become a channel for the arts, a state of being which is both profoundly ecstatic and acutely painful, often at the same time.

All great stories exist because of Her blessings, whether they take the form of a movie, a book, or a story related on some dark and lonesome night around a campfire. Her power is what brings it all together and makes it work, what makes it more than mere images on canvas or film or just an assortment of words upon a page. Her power provides the spark and flash that takes it that extra step. Her power is the glittering sprinkle of pixie dust which brings it to life.

Whenever a book or a movie or a story or a piece of art has had an profound effect on you, when it has touched your emotions or changed your life, then you have felt the touch of the Muse and seen Her art at work. She makes the magick which rouses millions, which inspires images and ideas that can alter the world for good or for ill. Without Her blessing, without Her influence—and those artists involved being open to that touch—it may be a good book or a decent enough movie, but it will never be *brilliant*. It will never become a living, breathing part of this reality. It will remain just simple entertainment, a distraction of the moment.

Talent is, more than anything else, the ability to open yourself up to the Muse, to give yourself over to the usages of Her gift. When you allow Her to work through you, marvels, mystery, and magick can be brought into reality. Not that skill and practice don't count, of course, as does perseverance—what can be taught in classes or through books or practical experience—but without the blessings of the Muse they will never amount to something grand and wonderful. Because, to create art which can truly become a part of someone else and transform their lives, you need the Muse.

Despite the modern world's love affair with reason and logic, most people still end up changing their lives for the main part based on what they feel, rather than what they think. Emotion is key to transformation and without that key the lock can stubbornly refuse to open, trapping people in a prison of their own thoughts, whether they are essentially good or sadly misguided. We all need a strong foundation to build upon, but we also need to remain flexible and emotion plays a powerful part in that.

Our lives are made up of patterns and habits that are both positive and negative, most of which have been laid down by conscious and unconscious feelings over the years. A lot of them were born out of our childhood, some from even before we could walk or talk. These patterns were deeply engrained into our minds and bodies, so much so that sometimes we can't even see them for ourselves. So to affect people, to really aid in a proper, quite often necessary transformative process, you have get down there and really touch their feelings. You have to get inside them and move them, help break the hold of old and probably outworn patterns, or at least serve to inspire them to examine their lives and see what should be changed. All of which requires the Muse.

Without the influence of the Muse, without that emotional rush, that intensity, that dreadful beat of bliss and terror, life can easily end up flat and unappealing. Sure, feelings and experiences like that can be scary, but what is the alternative? A world where there's no height of excitement anymore, no real pleasure, no bright colors, no sharp scents, no perfume of life or joy in sex or creation or in pursuing or fighting for anything. Without the power of inspiration and of the arts, what remains before you can easily slip into just one grey, empty day after another, month after month, year after year, not really living, not really feeling. Worst of all, not really knowing what life and love can be if you but gave yourself over to the full experience of them.

Of course, where there are heights there are also depths, as where there are peaks there are valleys. The valley of the shadow of depression, fear, doubt, and of empty disregard for all life can and should be. The modern world's tendency to rely on and run screaming to anti-depressants, with its focus on muting painful emotions so that mere "functionality" is achieved, runs the risk of disregarding and denigrating what the Muse has to offer us. Life just hurts too much sometimes so we give into the idea and the "cure" of being drugged into a reality where there are no real highs and no real lows left anymore. Where we're told over and over again that buying and owning things can make us feel better and productive.

Sadly, though, this *is* the wasteland. A world where order must rule at all costs, where mere physical objects are supposed to give our lives joy and meaning, where we tumble further and further from each other, so that we no longer know our neighbors, let alone share in any kind of real community and where illusions of safety, security, and surety are worth giving up every freedom for. And where people long for something special in their lives, something incredible, something to make them feel alive again. It may seem as though we in Western society today have a lot, especially when compared to our ancestors, but are we really any happier or more content than they?

What is this pain, this heartache, this wasteland, this darkness, this longing? It's the pain of a King who has forgotten himself, just as we have forgotten ourselves and where we first came from. It's the pain of living within the bounds of a desert-born religion which was never really ours to begin with nor ever really could be entirely, because its symbols were not born where we were born, anymore than its Gods were. Of course, some symbols are universal and all religions can lead you to the Divine so long as you don't get caught up in their dogma and lose the faith and meaning behind the stories…but we respond best to our *own* stories, to our *own* symbols, to our *own* heritage. To that which slumbers in our flesh and bone and blood—the world of the great forests of old, the woods and waters of our ancestors, and the glittering treasure which lies beneath the hill of Kings, the hill where Earth and sky meet and are made one. This is the world where the Muse lives still, where the Lady of the Lake keeps vigil over the sword of Kings.

For the past 2000 years, the Age of Pisces which is now passing away, She gave freely of Her services, allowing us to dip into the well of inspiration without asking permission and without even having to give our thanks to Her. To add insult to injury, She has also been defamed by some of the world's religions—as, in general, the vast majority of Goddesses from many cultures and times have been defamed or relegated to a lesser role—or even portrayed as ugly or wicked or terrible, as a demon or wanton whose very existence would drive otherwise righteous men to sin.

But for the Age of Aquarius, the Age of the Water-Bearer, inspiration will now come with a price tag...a price tag which is long overdue. For the next 2000 years, the Muse will *need* to be acknowledged and thanked for what She does for us. We will need to show our appreciation for the gifts that She bestows and ask for Her blessing on the arts that we pursue. Whenever we do anything well, whenever we do anything that is truly beautiful and magnificent, a gift that simply seems to flow out of us from somewhere else, then that is the work and blessing of the Muse and She will now need to be acknowledged for it. Otherwise, it is within Her prerogative to take it away.

It's a small thing to ask, really, to give thanks where thanks are due, especially considering we have been given what amounts to a "free ride" for the past twenty centuries. Not only that, but if the great leaps in the arts and sciences during the Renaissance Period came about *without* Her direct blessing then how much more can we accomplish and create if we engage in a living and viable relationship with Her? The Earth could truly become a jewel in the heavens if we turned our time and attention to beauty and the arts, all of us doing the best we can and being the best we can in all that we do.

We are the ones who can stand up and say no more. We are the ones who can transform the wasteland, learning to live this life to its fullest extent and regretting nothing at the end of our days. We are the ones who can learn to feel again, to find the Grail of our hearts and be King of our own destiny. One step along the way is to reclaim the Muse and Her powers of fantasy, daring, and wild creation.

Below is a prayer which can be used to ask Ariadne, otherwise known as the Lady of the Lake, Aphrodite, and the Muse for Her blessings on your life and art, whatever form that art takes:

a Prayer to the Muse

Oh beauteous one
To thee I pray,
Grant to me a taste of inspiration,
To drink of the cup
Of mind and heart and voice
Sealed to the arts
By your own immortal hand,
Your pledge and trust.
Grant to me such wonders
As yet unknown to man,
Pleasure beyond terror,
Dark and daring,
Truth and light,
Boundless of vision
And creative of delight.
Lend to me such spirits
As I may come to know your face
In every aspiration,
In each and every grace.

What is beauty, really, but a way to notice the Divine in the world around us, as well as in each other. The path of the Muse can be a way to bring more of the Divine into our lives, to acknowledge and express it. What is beauty but being thrown out of the sometimes humdrum and everyday blahs that we can fall in to if we're not careful and without even really wanting to. What is beauty but the ability to be shocked back to an awareness of the tragedy and comedy, the sheer beauty and sorrow of life, as they intermingle and constantly transform each other.

When you are confronted by something truly wonderful—and equally by something truly terrible—it opens you up inside. It unlocks the door, if only for a moment, and shocks you awake. After a time, the feeling fades and eventually loses its impact, but maybe, just maybe, some of its effects may linger a little, hopefully enough to keep you from rolling over and just going back to sleep. The more that this happens and the greater the impact, the greater the likelihood that you will remain awake in the world and be alive to the life that you life.

The power of the Muse can feel in some respects like falling in love, when everything and everyone around you suddenly becomes special and beautiful, as if your eyes were suddenly opened to a world you had all but forgotten about. Rose-colored glasses haven't been put over your eyes, making you see a world of lovely illusion, but instead it's as if the dank and murky lenses you were wearing before had abruptly fallen away, revealing the real world at long last. A world of breathless despair and hope, of bright promise and anguish...the world of the Muse.

If beauty is the rose of love then inspiration is the drink of the Divine. It's the sparkling, glimmering liquid that lies within the cauldron of Cerridwen, the one that makes the whole world shine. As it makes the entire web of life shine, the web She knows in Her aspect as Ariadne, mistress of spiders. For She *is* the lady of the dark cauldron, the cauldron which inspires all who drink from it. She is the rich and creamy sea-foam Goddess, Aphrodite, who rose from the waters of life and fertility. As well as being the Priestess-queen who once upon a time graced the King of the Land with a sword which was his own Divine nature made manifest. For the Muse, more than anything, once served to create the dream of Camelot, the shining city upon the shining hill.

We all have in within ourselves to drink from that cauldron, to know Her hand at work within ourselves, and to let ourselves be driven by that fierce creative force. Some people find it easier than others to give up control and simply trust, to let Her currents flow through them. Some people find it hard to give up control and just relax and let it go. Half the battle in some ways can be in finding your calling, in finding what it is that makes you *want* to surrender control and go with the bliss of creativity. The other half lies in persuading yourself that it's okay to do so, especially if things don't make a whole lot of sense at first or if society at large frowns upon what you want to do.

For example, if you have worked retail jobs your whole life and deep inside you there has always remained a burning dream of being a painter or an actor, then if you turn aside to purse that calling there may be those who will scoff at the thought. They might tell you that you are too old, that it's too late to go chasing after some pipedream. That you have to be practical or that what you want is simply too hard to do, that it's better not to try at all than to try and fail. But it's never too late, not for something that you well and truly desire beyond everything else, something that is your heart's true bliss.

This is not to say that it will come easy, especially if you are constantly being undermined by your own doubts or the doubts of others, but we can, if we but believe in it absolutely, do whatever we make up our hearts and minds to really do. It may look, afterwards, to some of those in the outside world like some sort of miracle or magick or "lucky break" took place, but it will have come from your own sense of self and that's what it actually made it happen for you. It will happen when you follow that love and make it your own, and work like hell to bring it into being in the world.

Unfortunately, though, one problem is that a lot of people today have a rather narrow definition of what the arts really are. Writing, painting, singing, photography, cooking, dancing, acting, all of these sorts of pursuits spring naturally to mind when you think of the arts. But they're just more obvious and not everyone will find their vocation leading them to do the obvious. For making love can be an art, as can wrapping gifts, farming, swimming, throwing parties, healing, giving massages, tours, and advice, among many other things. All of these can be an art so long as it brings something wonderful and beautiful into the world and serves to brighten people's hearts. Doubly so, if it also inspires someone else to go after their own bliss, to make the wasteland inside them blossom and bloom.

For we are not meant to live in the wasteland. We are meant to remember the secret of the Grail that opens the door to our own hearts and power. Functional does not mean alive. Functional means surviving, but what then are we surviving for without that knowledge? Without knowing what life is. Without waking up the King, who lives in each of us. The King who knows that he and the land are one, that what you believe in and what you create are one, that the inner world and the outer world are one.

In order to transform your life and bring about your own personal Camelot, you need to start there, inside yourself. To remember the secret of life and to reclaim the treasures that were yours to begin with. To dare to embrace the power of the Muse and of the arts, especially the art of life. For life means creation as it means emotion. It means daring to truly feel and be alive, even though that can be scary sometimes.

Our lives are our stories, they are our song, they are our drama play, and when you follow your heart and pursue your dreams, never giving up, never letting even your own doubts stop you, and keeping that dream as pure and bright as possible…then you are drinking from the cup of inspiration, the cup of immortality, the cup of life. You have found the cauldron, the one which provides what each of us needs the most.

We all have to find our own Grail, the dream and drink which will heal the wasteland and revive the King sleeping within the circle of our hearts. Especially at this time, at the dawn of a new Age, we each have to awaken and greet that golden light with a light of our own. A dull and grey world of unending drudgery is not the natural state of humankind, and certainly never the natural state of Witchkind. For life is meant to be hot and sharp, not bland and subdued. It's meant to have its ups and downs, not to exist in some middle place of nothing too much and never enough.

It may not always be easy, but life is meant to be lived.

The Good Game and Beyond

Dawn is the Gate of Life, the star of the East, the voice that first gave form to the world of men.

Dusk is the Gate of Death, the evening star, from whence dreams come to the hearts of men.

Between the Gates of Life and Death, between the pillars of dusk and dawn, lies the path of the wise. The path that leads to the realms beyond and to the beginning place which is the eternal source.

The middle path is that which lies between the light pillar and the dark, that which takes you there and back again.

But first there is the game.

I was lying in bed, somewhere in that pleasant world half way between being awake and being asleep, when the words "Benevento," "Blockula," "Venusburg" rang through my head. I felt weird, as though there were lots of strange energies running through my head and my body, as though I was vibrating fast and faster, as though something was just about to happen.

Just then, though part of me could still feel that I was lying in my bed, at the same time I felt like I was somewhere else entirely. The place that I saw had a kind of grayish-silver sky to it, one with no sun and no moon. There was a meadow of tall grass surrounded by trees, and it all looked silver-grey, too, almost as if a silver wash had been painted over green.

At first, the meadow appeared empty, but then a structure suddenly appeared at the far end. It kept changing through, as if it couldn't make up its mind what it wanted to be. At first, it looked like a sort of big hall, then it became a square castle with a round tower at each corner. At first there were no flags on the towers, but even as that thought went through my mind, there suddenly appeared all sorts of blue and green and yellow flags.

One moment I was in the meadow, looking at the flags on the castle, then I was suddenly inside that same structure. There was a big open hall full of people and I got the intense feeling that they had been expecting me. Or, rather, that they had been hoping to be able to expect me. Overall, the feeling at that moment was one of homecoming, though it was tinged with both happiness and sadness—sadness because it had taken so long, that we had been so long apart, and happiness because we were all together at last.

At the same time, I felt this sharp wave of emotion, as though I had somehow found some missing part of myself that I loved desperately. It'd been a test to get here and those who had waited for me to pass the test were now relieved and exulted and fulfilled, as much as I now felt relieved and exulted and fulfilled. To finally be home…

Then it all changed again and I was back outside and the structure was gone again. Instead, the meadow looked larger than before and there were two lines of people facing each other across its vast expanse. Everyone was riding on something, some sort of animal or bird mostly and a wind had picked up, the kind of wind which presages a coming storm. I was riding on a big crow and I felt strong and almost giddy with the wild energy building up in the meadow. Suddenly, both lines rushed right at each other and we ended up in a big, grand and glorious free-for-all, with everyone bashing good-naturedly at each other and screaming and generally having a high old time.

This, then, was Benevento. This, then, was the Witches' Sabbat. A place where sometimes you fEasted and sometimes you fought and sometimes you danced, each according to its own cycle and season and need. It felt very much like a Witch place, a place by and for Witches. Just as it felt real and not real at the same time, as if it both existed in and out of the world.

What you see is what you get…we've all heard that phrase. But when it comes to Benevento, it's more like what you get is what you see. What you expect to see, what you most need to see, is what you will end up seeing and experiencing. So if it is Benevento to you then it will *be* Benevento and if it is not, then it won't be. Which may sound like a riddle, but then we all know how much those of Faery like their riddles and this is as much a Faery place as it is a Witch place.

So when you travel to Benevento, to the Witches' Sabbat, what you'll end up experiencing there will be a combination of what you desire to see, what you require to see, and what the Game desires and requires of you to see. Though certain fundamental themes remain, themes that are deeply engrained in us and in our shared spiritual heritage as sons and daughters of the Old Ones. The patterns and symbols which run through the stories of Blockula, Venusburg, Josephat, Benevento, are ones that those of us of European descent, those of us who share the European soul, will be instinctually familiar with.

So we are drawn to the field, to the smell of flowers, and come to see a structure of some kind, as well as a well or a spring, one quite often near a tree. The tree itself may be a walnut tree, or an oak, a willow, a rowan, an ash, all of them a world trees, Faery trees, trees which span all ages and all worlds. We see a great house or a grand castle, the home of lords and ladies, of kings and queens, representing the idea and pledge of a noble line, of noble blood, of families who are linked to the land and are obligated to stewardship of that land and those who live upon it. While the flowers that we smell turn out to be wild roses, blushing pink in color, and with only five petals, a link to the five-pointed star of the Craft .

This is the Witches' crossroads, the star which is a heart which is a rose, and the field of battle, the hall of feasting, and the well and the tree…how could we really forget any of those? How could we forget what it is to ride into battle upon the back of your totem, the symbol of your power and secret inner nature? How could we forget the battle which is also a game which is also a dance, deadly serious and impossibly silly at the same time? As we fight and fEast and rise to fight again, the powers swirling around us, changing possibility, changing worlds, changing reality.

We play the Game to effect change. One world is altered and this, in turn, has an effect on another. It spreads out from there, each world altering the next. The Witches' Sabbat creates the first ripple as the Game is the stone thrown into still water, into the well of Benevento. Just as when we transform the Earth physically and spiritually, we transform what the Earth touches, whether that is ourselves or other worlds Seen and Unseen.

Because nothing is truly separate from anything else. All worlds are tied together in the web of Destiny.

Great changes move like storms across worlds, sometimes starting in one place, sometimes another…but all have their beginnings in Benevento, in the Game. We can't stop the storms when they come, but we can control how we react to them, whether we embrace change or attempt to forestall or flee from it. As individuals and as a people, humankind will transform from the Age of Pisces to the Age of Aquarius, but it remains in our hands, and in the hands of the worlds' Witches, just how this change will go. Whether it will happen in joy and with acceptance or whether people must be dragged kicking and screaming into the new paradigm.

Either way, it *will* happen, there's no way around it. The better choice, though, is to go with the flow and make the changes as peaceable and painless as possible. By riding the wave rather than being merely sucked along by the current, you stand far less risk of drowning. Just as any revolution that's necessary will happen eventually, the change of the Age is here and now, happening all around us. If people accept it a bit at a time and by their acceptance inspire others to accept it, then it can happen gently, without recourse to flame and chaos. It needn't reach the flashpoint of violence and destruction, but instead can be a long, patient process.

However, if the majority of people play games of denial, drag their feet and insist on going whistling blindly past the graveyard of the Piscean paradigm—or if they become more and more controlling in an effort to keep what they have, what they know, the institutions that they have built upon the back of the old Age—then it can and will end up in bloody revolution. It will end up in the hands of Tahlshai, Libertas, the Goddess of freedom. For She is both a lady of peace and of terror; it's our choice to decide what face we wish Her to wear on our behalf at this critical time.

What Witches can do to help turn the Age is to be both an example of the virtues of the next Age and to play the Game of Benevento. Witches need to be the vanguard, those who forge ahead and light the way forward for those who will follow. They need to bear up the standard of the Water-Bearer, the Star with Her cup pouring forth knowledge in equal measure upon both land and sea, the body and the spirit, this world and the world of Other.

To play the Game is to know yourself. To play the Game is to know the world. To play the Game and yet know it for a game—that is the true trick of it, the mark of a Witch of the old ways. For only then will you be able to go past the Game. Only then will you find yourself upon the road of eight, soaring past the four towers, past all that you have seen and all that you have felt and all that you know…going beyond the dream, beyond what is, and into what might yet be.

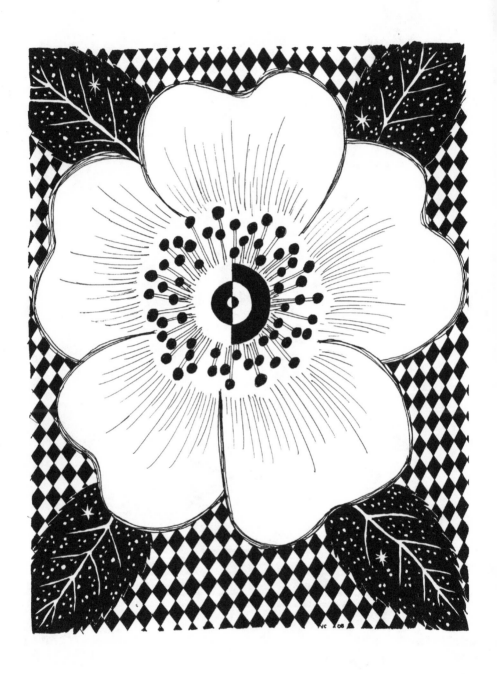

Conclusion

It is the purpose of Priests and Priestesses to call up and control Fate, to choose. Faith with choice is no longer faith, but knowledge.

Sahlonshai, Goddess of the South

What is it that we know about Witches then, especially those Witches who wish to renew the Blood, to come again into the full power and knowledge of the Old Ones?

We must wake the Blood. We must stir up the Blood so that it will remember. We must reclaim our history and our heritage, including our culture and language. We must take up the path of service to the community, to the Earth, and to the Gods. We must take the steps to find our way to Benevento, to the Witches' sacred Sabbat place of old, and there to play the Game. And, finally—though "finally" is a misnomer for there is no end and no last thing to do—we must go beyond the Game, all the way back to the Source, and return with gifts, with what is most needed in this time and in this place.

We are all on a Quest. A Quest to remember and to find the eternal spark within, that which makes us who we are.

We're not alone in this. We don't have to walk this path alone. Other Witches, both those here in the flesh and those yet in spirit form, including those Witches we once were and may yet be, they go with us, they stand with us. Other aspects of our Higher Spirits are also here for us, those brothers and sisters of the soul scattered across the universe. Not to forget, various familiar and strange elemental beings, our animal kin, and those of the Gods who hold us near and dear—all who travel with us, giving aid and

305

advice so that we may find the door and walk through it, the door to what the Craft really is all about.

The door by and to and for love.

But as this book is no more than words upon a page, it can only be a beacon, a guidepost, a spark to hopefully raise a fire. It remains to each Witch to dare to open the door into other realms, into the land of spirits, Gods, magick, and those secret and hidden powers that sleep and stir and desire to wake deep within us all.

It's my own fondest desire, wish, and hope that some few of these words, that some shining poetry hidden in them here and there, may find the means and measure to do just that…but that's not up to me. It's up to the Gods, Goddesses, and spirits who gave me these words, and to you yourself, to believe or not to believe, to have faith or not to have faith. It's your choice, as always, whether to open up your heart or keep it forever closed and locked away from the world.

These are all choices that each of us must make, for the gift of choice is one the greatest gifts ever given to us by the Divine essence. We each must make our own decisions, walk our own path, find our own way. Though, sometimes, if we are lucky and work very hard and seek the truth— both within us and without—we can find a few guides and companions, companions who share a common faith, resolve, and dream and guides who can give us hints and help along the way.

There are other gifts, of course. Some of which we have already, but don't know how to fully bring them into our lives. While others lie fallow, all but ignored, almost forgotten. Even as other gifts remain somewhere *out there*, past the last haunted peak of the Witches' Mountain, past the game of Benevento…there in the uncharted seas of the Beyond, where they wait for us to find them and bring them back here. To bring them home again.

Wake and do not forget.

Index

A

B

ecstasy 130
Elysian Fields 56
Eohvay 144, 145, 146
Eohvay, Invocation of 145

F

Faery 35, 95, 96, 236, 237, 238, 300
Faery Queen 96
family 21
fertility 106
Fey 8, 11, 95, 234, 236, 238, 239
Fire 102, 103, 104, 242, 243
fire 69
For All to Journey to Benevento 194
forge 103
For the Men to Journey into the Overworld 188
For the Women to Journey to the Underworld 182

G

Game 278
Game, the 59, 60, 61, 62, 278, 300, 302
Gate of Faery 94
Gate of the Gods 87
Gehhest 120, 121
Gehhest, Invocation of 121
Giahna 142, 143, 144, 146
Giahna, Invocation of 143
Glamour 233
glamour 232
Glamourie 230
glamourie 231
Gobah 227
Goddess 50
Goddess Invocation 161
God Invocation 162
Grail 125, 297
Guardian at the Gate 269
Guenivere 274
Guided Meditation to the Old Forest 180
Gwenhyvar 125, 126, 127, 244
Gwenhyvar, Invocation of 126

H

Hehren 114, 115, 243
Hehren, Invocation of 115
Hekahteh 136, 137, 138, 244
Hekahteh, Invocation of 137

Horn of Plenty 225

I

illuminare 103
Imbolc 105, 107, 242
incense 166

K

King 292
King's 85
King Oaks 75
Kings 71
Kingship 106
knot 223
Knot Charm 223
knots 222

L

Lady of the Lake 111, 294
Lady of the Quest 125
Lady of the Well 274
lamia 149
Lammas 88, 91, 242
Land, the 208
Lord of the Beasts 138
Lord of the Hunt 204

M

Magestar 152
Magestar, Invocation of 152
Magestrar 150, 151
Magicians 43
magick 30, 38, 45, 110, 230, 264
May Day 239, 242
Melusine 148, 149, 150
Melusine, Invocation of 149
Midsummer 85, 88, 107, 242, 243
Midwinter 85, 91, 105
Morgah 131, 132, 133, 244
Morgah, Invocation of 131
morning star 85
Mother 47
Mount Olympus 13, 56
Muse 291, 293, 295

N

W

Y

Available From Pendraig

Witchcraft
BALKAN TRADITIONAL WITCHCRAFT Radomir Ristic
HEDGERIDER Eric De Vries
MY CROOKED PATH Peter Paddon
THE CROOKED PATH Peter Paddon
THE FLAMING CIRCLE Robin Artisson
THE FORGE OF TUBAL CAIN Ann Finnin
THE HORN OF EVENWOOD Robin Artisson
THE PENDULUM Raven Womack

Ancient Egypt
ANCIENT EGYPTIAN MYSTERIES Peter Paddon

Wortcunning
AULDS AND ENTS Raven Womack
THE CROOKED PATH HERBAL Raven Womack
THE RAVEN'S FLIGHT BOOK OF INCENSE, OILS, POTIONS &
BREWS Raven Womack
THE WORTCUNNER'S WAY Raven Womack

Holistic Therapy
ANATOMY FOR HOLISTIC THERAPISTS Dr. Colin Paddon

www.pendraigpublishing.com

CPSIA information can be obtained
at www.ICGtesting.com
Printed in the USA
BVHW030019080321
601969BV00001B/19